Mindful Strategies for Adult Clients with Adverse Childhood Experiences

A Resource for Mind/Body Professionals

According to the National Institutes of Health, "mind and body practices generally have good safety records when done properly by a trained professional or taught by a well-qualified instructor. However, just because a practice is safe for most people doesn't necessarily mean it's safe for you."

"Your medical conditions or other special circumstances (such as pregnancy) may affect the safety of a mind and body practice. When considering mind and body practices, ask about the training and experience of the practitioner or teacher, and talk with that person about your individual needs. Also, don't use a mind and body practice to postpone seeing a health care provider about a health problem" (Mind and Body Practices, 2017).

ISBN-13: 978-1-7328066-7-2

ISBN: 1-7328066-7-5

CONTENTS

IMPORTANT NOTES:

Research studies, published literature on mindfulness, expert perspectives, and client testimonies were used to compile the tips discussed in this book.

Keep in mind that some experts may disagree and scientific advances may render some of this information outdated. The author assumes no responsibility for any outcome based on the information shared in this book for self-care. If you have safety questions about the application of techniques discussed in this book, please consult your physician or mental health provider.

Quick Start Guide

FOREWORD

We are all products of our childhood experiences, and as such, most of us have experienced some degree of childhood adversity—even if we do not fully recognize it. The truth is even the slightest childhood trauma can affect us as adults.

Unbeknownst to many, almost all mental health conditions, including anxiety, depression, post-traumatic-stress disorder (PTSD), obsessive-compulsive disorder (OCD), panic attacks or panic disorder, attention-deficit hyperactivity disorder (ADHD), substance abuse, and addiction stem from adverse childhood experiences or ACEs. ACEs can imprint on a child's brain manifesting emotionally, socially, sexually, and/or physically later in life—years or decades after the traumatic event.

So, what is the best way to heal the deep wounds of ACEs and build strength and resilience in clients who are grappling with high levels of stress, caused by chronic conditions?

In this innovative book, Kathleen Lisson, lymphedema therapist, presents practical, evidence-based mindful strategies that mental health providers, health coaches, and therapists can use to help their clients heal from ACEs. In addition to dealing with the symptoms, providers can learn how to address the root cause of their clients' suffering, change the way their brains respond to stress and the outside world, and reduce or eliminate upsetting memories.

As a child and family psychologist with over 15 years of experience and a chronic illness, I can honestly say that I learned a lot from reading this book. It is important to understand that one of the most prevalent byproducts of having a chronic illness is stress. Stress can impact a chronically ill person's life in many ways, such as self-esteem and self-confidence, problem solving abilities, social interactions, coping mechanisms, and health and well-being.

When you add-in other childhood adversities, you have a recipe for lifelong mental health issues. The good news is there is a way to help adults who experienced ACEs heal and thrive.

Kathleen Lisson has provided clear explanations, scientific evidence, and actionable steps to help you provide the best care for your clients. This book provides the key to reaching clients, who have built a wall to protect themselves from further harm. It is a book that I plan to use in my own practice because I truly believe it can make a difference in the lives of my clients.

Dr. R.Y. Langham

(Child & Family Psychologist)

INTRODUCTION

"You may not control all the events that happen to you, but you can decide not to be reduced by them."
~Maya Angelou

"I am convinced that the great mass of our people go through life without even a glimmer of what they could have contributed to their fellow human beings. This is a personal tragedy. It is a social crime. The flowering of each individual's personality and talents is the precondition for everyone's development."
~James Reid

The inspiration for this book is the result of conversations that I have had with a client with lipedema who came to me for manual lymphatic drainage. This client is a survivor of adverse childhood experiences (or ACEs) that happened when she was a child in post–World War II England.

My client has spent the last few years coming to terms with the emotional roots of her chronic illnesses by learning from experts like Gabor Mate. She found the combination of full-body manual lymphatic drainage sessions and a safe space to feel her emotions very healing. I did not verbally respond to or counsel her, I simply listened to her recount her childhood experiences.

My client's account of how stress has affected her chronic illness is not unique. In fact, Buck and Herbst state that women with lipedema can experience rapid growth of the lipedema subcutaneous adipose tissue when confronted with stress, surgery, and/or hormonal changes (Buck & Herbst, 2016).

Lipedema is not the only disease that is affected by stress. In the article, "Stress and Chronic Illness: The Inflammatory Pathway," Acabchuk et al. found that "social adversity" can get under a person's skin through their immune system, and that the link between social disadvantage and chronic illness is reconciled in part by changes in immune cell distribution. The researchers also found that chronic inflammation is a major contributor in almost all of today's chronic diseases (Acabchuk et al., 2017).

Mind / body professionals who feel drawn to help others, whether we are counselors, family support partners, health coaches, massage therapists, meditation teachers, occupational therapists, personal trainers, peer support, physical therapists, promotoras, psychologists or yoga instructors, can create a "safe space" for clients, who deserve to be introduced to new treatments, tools, and techniques that can lower their stress levels. Self-awareness and increased confidence, along with new mindfulness skills, can encourage clients to gently set aside unhealthy "numbing" coping mechanisms, in favor of healthier ways of coping with life's stressors.

Why is understanding these skills so important?

Dr. Perry states in his book, *What Happened to You?* that without some degree of regulation, it can be hard to fully connect with someone else, and without a connection, there is limited reasoning. Thus, trying to reason with someone before they are "balanced" will not work, and will only worsen frustration (dysregulation) for everyone involved (Perry & Winfrey, 2021).

The first step?

Learning what the research says about adverse childhood experiences and how toxic stress affects the mind and body.

The next step?

Exploring mindfulness exercises that may boost our clients' resiliencies and help them *bounce forward*, instead of *backward* after experiencing adversity.

In the words of trauma professional David A. Treleaven, "resilience increases our capacity to be present with life as it is" and "by helping survivors be strategic with their attention, we can help them utilize mindfulness to find stability in the midst of traumatic symptoms" (2018).

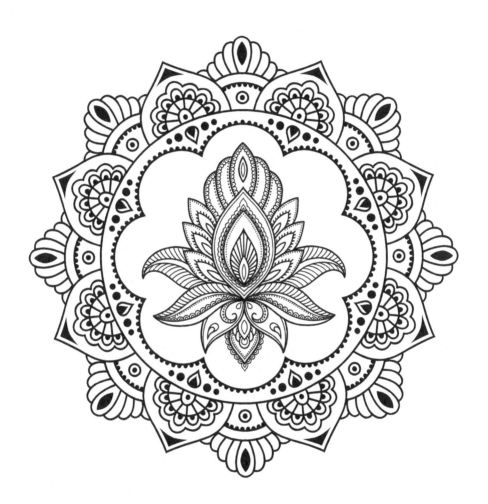

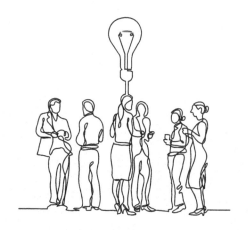

CHAPTER 1

WHAT ARE ADVERSE CHILDHOOD EXPERIENCES?

What helped my client better understand herself and what inspired her to continue the hard work of daily self-care for her chronic disease? She learned about a type of trauma called adverse childhood experiences (ACEs).

According to the ACEs Aware Trauma-Informed Network of Care Roadmap, ACEs are traumatic events that occur during childhood.

More specifically, the term ACEs refers to ten categories of adversity in three domains – abuse, neglect, and household challenges - that are experienced before the age of eighteen (ACEs Aware Trauma-Informed Network of Care Roadmap, 2021).

Listed below are the "adverse childhood experiences" researched in the landmark CDC-Kaiser Permanente study published in 1998.

- Physical abuse
- Emotional abuse
- Sexual abuse
- Physical neglect
- Emotional neglect
- Domestic violence
- Addiction
- Mental illness
- Incarceration
- Divorce or parental separation

These are stressful situations, especially for a child's growing brain. Their little bodies are seeking safety and not finding it. When the body's stress response remains activated for a long period, the result is increased inflammation and hormone disruption. Also, when a child chronically experiences this kind of stress, it affects their brain development. Research has shown that an adult with one or more unmitigated ACEs has an increased risk for multiple chronic diseases.

Which diseases?

According to the article, "The Role of Mindfulness in Reducing the Adverse Effects of Childhood Stress and Trauma," these diseases include mental health disorders, adult ischemic heart disease, cancer, chronic lung disease, skeletal fractures, and liver disease (Ortiz & Sibinga, 2017).

What are the mitigating factors?

Children experiencing ACEs with at least one stable and supportive adult in their lives are less likely to experience toxic stress and develop unhealthy coping strategies that can lead to chronic diseases, as compared to those who do not have at least one stable and supportive adult in their lives.

Listed below is an example of a screening tool that includes questions about ACEs and the mitigating factors:

Threshold Global Works:

https://www.thresholdglobalworks.com/pdfs/PACES-with-provider-note.pdf

You can learn more about the concept of risk and protective factors here:

SAMHSA (the US government's Substance Abuse and Mental Health Services Administration): https://www.

samhsa.gov/sites/default/files/20190718-samhsa-risk-protective-factors.pdf

Do ACEs cause mental health disorders?

In the article, "Mindfulness: As a Mediator and Moderator in the Relationship Between Adverse Childhood Experiences and Depression," McKeen, et al. explain that ACEs *could* worsen adult mental health issues, partly due to changes in the structure and function of the body's stress-response systems (2021).

For instance, some people turn to substances like alcohol, tobacco, or other drugs to cope with stress. Thus, researchers suggest that there is a link between ACEs and mental health disorders and substance use disorders (MSUDs).

One such study, "Association of Adverse Childhood Experiences with Lifetime Mental and Substance Use Disorders Among Men and Women, Aged 50 Years Old," examined the relationship between ACEs and lifetime MSUDs in people over the age of fifty, and found that child abuse, parental mental illnesses, and substance abuse are significant predictors of MSUDs.

Researchers also found that six ACEs (e.g., the three types of child abuse, parental/other adult mental illnesses, parental/other adult substance abuse, and parental divorce) are positively correlated with one or more lifetime substance use disorders (Choi et al., 2016).

So as you can see, ACEs deliver a one-two punch. Experiencing toxic stress can have a negative effect on the body, and relying on unhealthy coping mechanisms to deal with the effects of trauma can lead to even more adverse effects.

Our goal should not be to use this information as a diagnostic or treatment tool. We are sharing information on ACEs and providing assistance, referrals, and resources to our clients. ACEs are not "conditions;" rather, they are "aspects" of a person's history (e.g., past experiences). We must be careful to not stigmatize the people we are trying to help.

How do ACEs function in the brain? More specifically, how does having ACEs affect a child's brain?

Stress and toxic stress can affect the body through an increased allostatic load; the physiologic burden of such stress may, in turn, manifest as "neuroanatomical changes," increased inflammation, and hypothalamic-pituitary-adrenal axis dysfunction. ACEs have also been linked to biological markers of disease, such as inflammatory cytokines, metabolic abnormalities, and epigenetic modifications (Ortiz & Sibinga, 2017).

What does this look like in real life?

Individuals with a history of ACEs may have an increased risk of developing a negative or unhealthy cognitive style that makes it hard to cope with life stressors. Researchers suggest that these individuals are more likely to have a negative perception of their environment (e.g., as posing greater and more numerous illogical threats and an increased likelihood of internalizing negative emotions) (McKeen et al., 2021).

The Bottom Line: Clients with ACEs may think that they are broken, but they are not. Their bodies are simply reacting to chronic levels of toxic stress. As a result, it is imperative that we encourage them to give themselves a break. They don't have to be so hard on themselves.

ACTION STEP

How can we introduce the concept of ACEs into our conversation with our clients?

Some clients already know their ACE score—for instance, they may have taken an NPR quiz, or been tested at their physician's office. Others may have never heard of ACEs or feel uncomfortable when remembering their childhood. Some may communicate about their childhood in a very matter of fact way and not think it affects them at all. I highly recommend ensuring that your clients feel a sense of safety *and* a connection to you *before* bringing up ACEs.

Perhaps, you can say, "Your body may be producing excessive stress hormones. Your past experiences may also be triggering your intrusive thoughts and/or feelings of shame, judgment, and self-blame. There are several ways we can reduce the effects of toxic stress on your body. Would you like to know more?"

"But first, I would like to know if you feel relatively safe right now."

This is an important question to ask.

Why?

Because we need to build trust with our clients first. Even though we will not be asking them to talk about their pasts, our clients need to be in a space, physically and mentally, where they can and are willing to confront tough issues. Thus, we, as professionals, must refrain from re-traumatizing our clients.

For instance, if a client says, "No, I do not feel safe right now" you can then ask them, "What will make you feel safe?" or "What has helped you feel safe in the past?" Emphasize that you are NOT asking them to share intimate details about their childhood. Also, explain to your client that the goal is to work together to help them more effectively manage their stress, as an adult.

Do not proceed until the client feels safe.

Let's look at a few more questions I have used in working with people with the chronic disease:

- "Would you be interested in developing skills to 'balance' your responses to your stressors?"

- "How do you manage your current health concerns?" (This question provides us with an opportunity to lead our clients—e.g., recognize their strengths, and enhance those strengths.).
- "What are some difficult experiences you have had to deal with in the past year because of your condition?
- "When I get to know you better, what qualities will I admire most about you?"
- "What do you think will happen if you continue to have severe symptoms in the next weeks and months?"
- "Have you sought guidance from another health professional? If so, what did they miss?" (This question provides us with an opportunity to listen to the client's unmet needs and tailor our responses, as needed.)
- "Would you like to get your health condition under control quickly, moderately, or gradually?"

We can support our clients' positive strengths, and encourage them to continue doing what is working for them in the self-care domains of:

- Mindfulness
- Physical activity
- Time in nature
- Positive relationships
- Sleep

Another great question is: *"Do you think stress is playing a role in your health issues? If so, how?"*

Our clients come to us because they care enough about themselves to seek our help. Self-care techniques and knowing their ACE scores can reassure these individuals that they are neither broken nor crazy, and they are by no means alone.

PARADIGM SHIFT

Why does recognizing ACEs in our clients matter?

It matters because it is common to expect that clients who come to us for help have certain life skills – when that may not be true.

We may expect clients to:

- Have an awareness and understanding of the world around them
- Understand the potential positive and negative consequences of their actions
- Know and feel their bodies
- Be able to effectively solve problems and plan for the future
- Recognize their feelings, learn from them, and effectively manage them
- Have the capacity for self-efficacy

- Be able to form trusting relationships, and trust and rely on the people in their lives

How does this look in real life?

People come to us because they are struggling with *something*—something they have not been able to solve by themselves or even with help from others.

If you suspect that a client has dismissed or ignored previous advice from a health professional or family member, or feel that the client simply does not care, you may do one or both of the following:

- Ignore or disregard the client's history of ACEs
- Provide the client with "solutions" based on the assumption that they have all of the necessary life skills, and simply lack motivation

Can you see how disregarding our client's history or jumping to providing 'cookie cutter' solutions will NOT serve our clients' needs?

Why can't we just try to boost our clients' motivation?

Listening to motivational content can inspire us for an hour or a day - but is motivation alone a reliable long term solution? Our clients may have coping strategies that may include anger, substance use, ignoring their own needs, and/or withdrawal from stressful situations.

- Do our 'solutions' require our clients to use 'motivation' to stop using current coping strategies used to ease their pain without offering alternative self-care tools?

- Are we requiring our client to "just get over it" and use 'motivation' to cope with the effects of their past traumas without offering alternative self-care tools?

PARADIGM SHIFT

Psychiatrist Bessel van der Kolk explains that people who rely on unhealthy or maladaptive coping mechanisms do not adopt them because they are lazy or unmotivated— they retain them because they are hard to give up. Unfortunately, little consideration is given to the possibility that many long-term health risks may be beneficial in the short-term (Van der Kolk, 2014).

Thus, if we ask our clients to stop relying on unhealthy or maladaptive coping strategies, we must also teach them beneficial stress-reduction skills that they can use in times of need. If our clients come to us for help with their behaviors—e.g., a behavior change, a specific coping strategy, etc., we should ask them, "What does this strategy solve?" and "What does it cost?"

ACTION STEP

Some people have "inner voices" that tell them that their reactions to trauma are just excuses. As a result, these individuals may judge themselves too harshly for feeling hurt, and truly believe that what happened to them was their fault—perhaps because of their laziness or because they are somehow bad. These individuals may also link needing and asking for help to self-coddling.

We can also ask, "Did this mindset help you accomplish your goals in the past? If not, are you open to trying something new?" Asking for permission *before* providing input was a large and important part of my training as a health coach; it is also good advice for interacting with clients with trauma histories.

Later in the book, we will learn more about the "inner voices" that accuse our clients of being "weak."

The Bottom Line: ACEs, along with accompanying stress responses and coping strategies, are NOT our client's faults. ACEs are risk factors, not grim predictors of our clients' destinys. The truth is that "this is not me; this is a result of something that *happened* to me."

Let's end this chapter with a moment of mindfulness.

Here is a mindfulness technique that can help you refocus and re-center:

The STOP Technique

Created by Jon Kabat-Zinn, the **STOP** technique is designed to get us off of "autopilot."

The steps are:

1. **Stop**: Stop what you are doing for a moment.
2. **Take a Breath**: Pay attention to the next breath you take.
3. **Observe**: What are you feeling at this moment? Do any bodily sensations stand out? You do not need to change or judge these sensations, only observe them.
4. **Proceed**: Return to what you were previously doing.

Later in the book, you will learn more about the STOP technique and other easy mindfulness techniques that can be added to your daily life.

Here are my original motivational interviewing questions for clients with lymphedema:

- "Would you be interested in developing skills that can help control your lymphedema?"
- "How do you manage your lymphedema symptoms now?"
- "Within the last year, what are some difficult lymphedema experiences you have had, and how did you deal with them?"

- "When I get to know you better, what qualities will I admire most about you?"
- "What do you think will happen if your lymphedema symptoms are not treated within the next few weeks or months?"
- "Have you sought guidance from another lymphedema expert? What did they miss?"
- "Would you like to quickly get your lymphedema under control?"

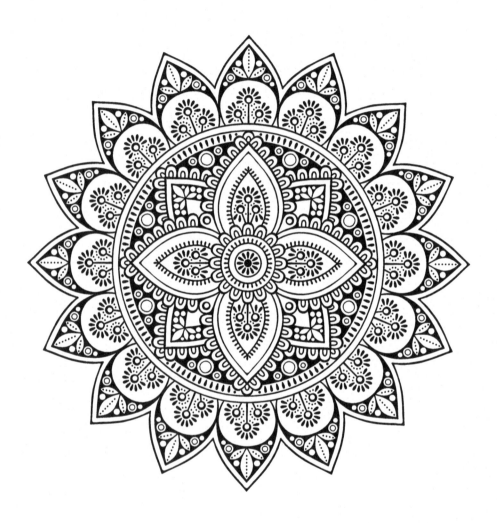

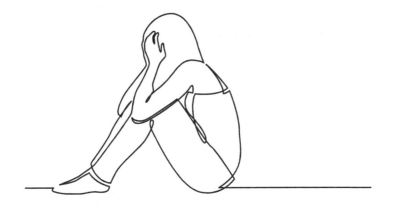

CHAPTER 2

WHAT IS TOXIC STRESS?

Everyone has felt stress in their life, and almost everyone has undergone a stressful life event.

How do ACEs affect our experiences of stress, and how does tolerable stress turn into toxic stress?

First, let's look at the different types of stress responses.

Positive stress

- A normal stress response
- Essential for growth and development
- Infrequent, short-lived, and mild
- Person is supported during stressful events

- Triggers motivation and resilience
- Involves biochemical reactions that can be returned to baseline once the stress eases

Tolerable stress

- Severe, frequent, and/or sustained stress response
- Involves responsive relationships and strong social and emotional support systems
- Involves biochemical responses that have the potential to negatively affect the brain's architecture
- Involves biochemical reactions that can be returned to baseline once the stress eases

Toxic stress

- Involves a prolonged activation of the stress response
- Involves a lack of support, reassurance, and/or emotional attachments
- Failure of the body to fully recover
- Results in increased vulnerability to maladaptive health outcomes (Franke, 2014)

Everyone has experienced positive stress at one time or another - taking a test, getting married, competing in an athletic event. Sports coaches excel at helping athletes perform under positive stress conditions. Our clients are going to come to us looking for help with tolerable or toxic stress, so let's look at the differences between them.

Tolerable Stress vs. Toxic Stress

According to the Harvard University Center on the Developing Child, a tolerable stress response activates the body's alert system due to severe, long-lasting adversities, such as the loss of a loved one, a natural disaster, or a frightening injury. If the activation is time-limited and buffered by relationships with adults who can help a child adapt to their new reality, their brain and other organs can recover from damaging effects (Toxic Stress, n.d.).

What can go wrong during toxic stress?

A toxic stress response typically occurs when a child experiences strong, frequent, and/or prolonged adversities, such as physical, sexual, and/or emotional abuse, chronic neglect, abandonment, caregiver substance abuse or mental illness, exposure to violence, and/or family economic hardship without adequate adult support.

What is the result?

This kind of prolonged stress response system activation can disrupt the development of brain architecture and other organ systems, and increase the risk for stress-related diseases and/or cognitive impairment well into the adult years (Toxic Stress, n.d.).

The presence or absence of a "trusted adult" who understands the child's situation and helps them adapt to it, is a significant difference between tolerable stress and toxic stress. Thus, the key to stopping ACEs is early intervention.

When I ask adults with chronic illnesses to raise their hands or comment if they were surrounded by trusted adults who consistently supported and understood them during childhood, only a few hands usually go up, and I only receive a few positive comments.

These are the people we are helping. So let's focus on toxic stress and a toxic stress response.

What is a toxic stress response?

A toxic stress response involves a prolonged or permanent abnormal physiologic response to a stressor with the risk of organ dysfunction. Childhood toxic stress involves severe, prolonged, and/or repetitive adversities that lack the necessary caregiver nurturance or support to prevent an abnormal stress response (Franke, 2014).

What happens to the body during toxic stress?

Prolonged cortisol activation and a persistent inflammatory state can cause the body to fail to "normalize" once the stressor has been eliminated. Thus, children who experience toxic stress are at risk of long-term adverse health effects, such as maladaptive coping skills, poor stress management, unhealthy lifestyles, mental illness, and physical disease (Franke, 2014).

What specifically causes toxic stress?

Toxic stress may stem from various situations, such as a single stressor that involves prolonged exposure (e.g., recurrent emotional abuse), multiple stressors that involve toxicity when aggregated (e.g., low socioeconomic status), poverty, having limited educational opportunities, and/or experiencing trauma of greater emotional intensity or severity (e.g., sexual abuse) (Ortiz & Sibinga, 2017).

What happens in our brains when we experience chronic stress?

Delude (2015) states that chronic stress can cause hippocampus neurons and the prefrontal cortex to shrink and lose their normal connections. This limits the brain's ability to transmit signals throughout the body via neurotransmitters that can help a child learn, remember information and events, solve problems, plan, and exercise self-control. During this time, the amygdala expands and becomes hypervigilant, sensing danger, anger, and sadness everywhere.

What is the result?

Your body accumulates fat and your immune system triggers chronic inflammation. Without normal regulation, your metabolic and appetite control systems trend towards overeating, insulin resistance, and diabetes, and your hippocampus has fewer glucocorticoid receptors—

receptors needed to turn off the stress response (Delude, 2015).

PARADIGM SHIFT

Wow! That certainly makes me realize how destructive toxic stress can be. However, we need *some* stress in our lives to grow. A "no-stress lifestyle" can lead to boredom and/or "laziness." A problem occurs when stress overwhelms our nervous systems. Chronic stress can negatively affect our bodies and brains.

Here are some questions we can ask ourselves about our own self-care:

- "What words do I say to myself, and what situations do I put myself in that trigger my stress responses?"
- "What types of out-of-control stressors do I experience?"
- "Do I tend to pre-plan and schedule self-care activities, doctors' appointments, home and car maintenance, or other tasks in advance? Or do I tend to wait until something breaks or breaks down, and then rush to get it fixed?"
- "Do I plan my meals in advance? Or do I tend to eat on the go?"
- "Do I typically foster responsive relationships and strong social and emotional support systems?"

- "How do I usually lower my stress level so I can recover from a stressful day?"

ACTION STEP

What steps can we take to balance our stress arousal levels?

For some, it could be a walk in the woods, while for others, it could be meditation. Both are great options! It is important to affirm the self-care steps our clients are already taking and encourage them to add more positive options to their stress-reduction toolboxes.

The Bottom Line: According the article, "Beginning the Healing Journey: Return to the Resilient Zone," Resilience Training International founder Glenn Schiraldi states that dysregulated or "unbalanced" stress arousal levels—arousal levels that are either too high or too low—are at the center of the ACEs' health outcomes.

That is, ACEs can lead to dysregulated stress, which in turn, can lead to stress-related symptoms. Thus, an important first step to healing the suffering caused by toxic childhood stress is to break the ACEs/health outcomes link by returning stress arousal to appropriate levels (Schiraldi, 2021).

Let's finish the chapter with a moment of mindfulness.

Deep Breathing and Soothing Touch

- Place your hand over your heart.
- Take a deep breath, while moving your hand in a soothing circular motion over your heart.
- Do this for at least 5 breaths, while repeating to yourself, "This is hard, but it will not be like this forever."

In the article, "Self-Soothing Touch and Being Hugged Can Reduce Cortisol Responses to Stress: A Randomized Controlled Trial on Stress, Physical Touch, and Social Identity," Dreisoerner et al. state that people who utilize "self-soothing touches" and who receive hugs have fewer cortisol secretion responses to socio-evaluative stress, and lower average cortisol values on three out of four measurement points after a stressful event. Moreover, the self-soothing touches appear to help people balance their cortisol levels faster than the control group (Dreisoerner et al., 2021).

The "soothing touch intervention" involves 20-seconds of self-soothing touches to calm oneself. Options include placing one or two hands on the heart or abdomen or stroking one's upper arms or cheeks. We should encourage our clients to choose a way to touch themselves that feels comfortable to them. Instruct your clients to take two or three deep breaths, and concentrate on the warmth, pressure of their hand(s), and breathing patterns.

Most people chose to place their right hand on the left sides of their chest (above their heart) with their left hand on their abdomen (Dreisoerner et al., 2021). Researchers have concluded that self-soothing touches are a highly effective way to reduce or eliminate the effects of pandemic stress (Dreisoerner et al., 2021).

How did you feel after this moment of mindfulness?

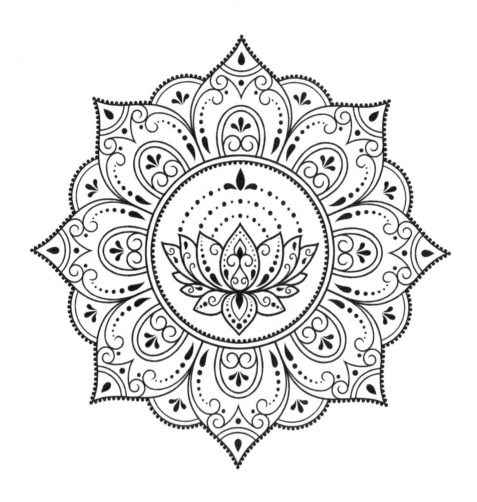

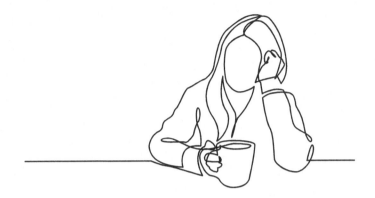

CHAPTER 3

THE ROLE OF STRESS REACTIVITY IN HELPING CLIENTS WITH BEHAVIOR CHANGE

We just learned from Glenn Schiraldi that dysregulated or uncontrolled stress arousal—arousal that is too high or too low—is at the center of the ACEs/health outcomes link (Schiraldi, 2021).

What is the relationship between dysregulated or uncontrolled stress response, stress reactivity, and addiction?

In the article, "Stress Reactivity and the Developmental Psychopathology of Adolescent Substance Use," Chaplin et al. state that stress reactivity involves perception, appraisal, and the response to harmful, threatening, and/or challenging events or stimuli.

According to researchers from George Mason University, in most cases, stress responses which stem from mild stressors (e.g., studying for a test) that can elicit a normative stress response in children, allowing them to harness mild negative emotions, and adaptively respond to these stressors (e.g., slight worry).

However, in some cases, children and adolescents may show a dysregulated or uncontrolled or "unbalanced" stress response, such as very high or very low/blunted reactivity to stress. These patterns may develop in children who have experienced repeated chronic and uncontrollable stressors (e.g., chronic child abuse, abandonment, or neglect; dysfunctional parenting; and/or chronic stressful environments, like living in dangerous neighborhoods) that have altered their stress reactivity systems (Chaplin et al., 2018).

This can become dangerous when children with blunted stress reactivity experience environmental stressors during adolescence and begin to exhibit poor emotional responses. To cope with poor arousal, some adolescents deliberately seek out illegal or addictive substances to control their emotions, and trigger positive emotions/sensations (Chaplin et al., 2018).

ACTION STEP

When our clients come to us for help setting goals around quitting alcohol or cigarettes or other addictive substances, consider sharing strategies that will help them regulate their stress reactivity.

How do we react to overwhelming feelings?

In the article, "9 Signs You Need Better Self-Care and May Be a Trauma Survivor," Robyn E. Brickel, MA, LMFT, asserts that trauma makes the inner world too uncomfortable and chaotic to have a curious awareness. Feeling alone with extreme fear and anxiety can trigger an urgent need to protect oneself from harm. So these individuals seek to "escape" overwhelming feelings because they are unable to safely explore them (Brickel, 2018).

How could trauma survivors "escape" these feelings?

Trauma survivors "escape" these feelings by learning to adapt. More specifically, these individuals develop responses that may *seem* like self-care, but are actually coping mechanisms. Coping often includes hiding your emotional needs not only from other people, but also from yourself. This helps you divert your attention, numb your feelings, or deny the emotional turmoil within (Brickel, 2018).

PARADIGM SHIFT

We've all heard someone recommend taking a few deep breaths, a walk, or a bubble bath. *Why don't people just use popular self-care tools to reduce their stress? Shouldn't this be common sense to our clients?*

The clients who would benefit the most from self-care tools may not believe they need or deserve them. We can make a difference if we understand this about our clients.

Trauma survivors often have trouble seeing and accepting their own self-care needs because:

- They do not like bringing attention to themselves, primarily because the inner world has been painfully overwhelming, or being seen by others was "risky" or "dangerous."
- They do not know how to trust the attention they are receiving from others because historically, attention has been abusive or negative.
- Their tolerance for pain and discomfort is high.
- They do not believe they deserve the good things life has to offer.
- They simply do not know how life *could* be different (Brickel, 2018).

ACTION STEP

How can we help our clients with trauma histories release their stress, if they do not trust the attention they are receiving, and/or if they have become accustomed to emotional dysregulation?

There are no super-secret techniques. Brickel suggests that trauma survivors should resort to trying healthy ways of releasing stress, like exercising, connecting with friends, meditating, practicing yoga, and/or journaling (Brickel, 2018).

Later in the book, we will talk more about these interventions.

This is where people who provide peer support and have lived experience can really make a positive difference! Interacting with people who regularly practice self-care, and can share how it has improved their lives, can be helpful for clients who are still on the fence as to whether self-care would work for them.

How do we react to intrusive, upsetting thoughts?

For some clients, stressors are the "gifts that keep on giving" long after the stressful incident has passed.

Let's look at two ways our thoughts can cause stress— the "inner critic" and rumination.

The "Inner Critic"

Do you have a critical voice in your head? You are not alone, and yes, it really can be your mother's voice you hear. According to the article, 'Dialogical Self Theory (DST),' human consciousness functions as a "society of mind," which involves mental representations of various cultural voices and voices of family members, close friends, significant others, etc. Some of these voices may be critical and judgmental (Oles et al., 2020).

There are different types of negative self-talk. Let's look at self-criticism and ruminative dialogues. Oles et al. state that self-criticism involves self-talk about aversive events (e.g., "I should have done that differently" or "I feel ashamed of what I did.").

Similar to self-criticism, ruminative dialogues involve self-blame, mulling over failures, and/or recalling sad or annoying thoughts or memories (e.g., "After failures, I blame my thoughts" or "I have confusing conversations in my mind") (Oles et al., 2020).

Let's learn more about rumination.

Rumination

What is rumination and why is it dangerous?

Rumination is defined as repetitive, unwanted, or intrusive thoughts. For individuals who ruminate, or mentally rehash past stressful events, the physiological effects of stressors can be long-lasting (Zoccola & Dickerson, 2012).

What is wrong with rehashing previous arguments or tense situations?

For people who dwell on arguments, elevated levels of stress hormones could continue to circulate in their bodies long after the argument has ended. Stress-related rumination is linked to increased cortisol concentrations and prolonged exposure to cortisol by the exaggerated, extended, or repeated activation of a maladaptive HPA axis.

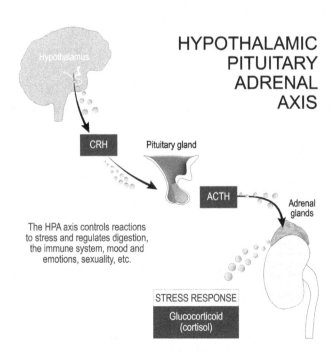

In fact, a variety of health conditions, including insulin resistance and cardiovascular disease, have been associated with persistent activation of the HPA axis (Zoccola & Dickerson, 2012). So ruminating on past incidents can cause the body to keep producing and releasing stress hormones like cortisol, even after the danger is gone.

Rumination, Pain-related Worry, & Nocebo Hyperalgesia

Feeling anxious as a pain symptom may actually have a role in increasing our clients' pain levels. "Pain catastrophizing" is characterized as a persistent pattern of distressing cognitive and emotional responses to current or anticipated pain (Darnall & Colloca, 2018).

"Catastrophizing" is seen as a pejorative term by many clients, so I prefer to use the term, "pain-related worry."

Pain-related worries may also include rumination (e.g., "I cannot stop thinking about how much it hurts."), magnification (e.g., "I worry that something bad will happen."), and/or "helplessness" (e.g., "There is nothing I can do to reduce my pain.") (Darnall et al., 2017).

Understand that your client's chronic and/or escalating pain is not just in their head.

In the article, "Nocebo Hyperalgesia: How Anxiety is Turned into Pain," Colloca & Benedetti state that negative pain expectations can worsen anticipatory anxiety geared towards chronic and/or escalating pain. The pain and anxiety can trigger the production of cholecystokinin, which in turn can worsen severe and/or chronic pain (Colloca & Benedetti, 2007).

What can we do to reduce the effects of rumination?

Mindfulness has been shown to protect against symptoms of psychological distress, such as depression, anxiety, and rumination (McKeen et al., 2021).

How does mindfulness work?

Mindfulness can reduce, limit, or prevent the consequences of toxic stress from repeated exposure to high-stress environments and can improve long-term coping skills, and accompanying physiologic effects of stress on the HPA axis (Ortiz & Sibinga, 2017). Mindfulness, with its focus on nonjudgmental acceptance, could help our clients learn how to cope better during stressful events.

Self-compassion may also reduce rumination. According to Frostadottir & Dorjee, self-compassionate people may experience lower levels of rumination and self-criticism.

Interestingly, these researchers recommend that mindfulness teachers refrain from explicitly discussing or teaching self-compassion during therapy. Instead, the researchers suggest that people learn these principles by watching the self-compassionate actions of mindfulness teachers. Additionally, researchers stated that "those experiencing higher levels of rumination may benefit from meditations focusing on mindfulness, whereas people with lower levels of rumination may benefit more from loving kindness practices" (Frostadottir & Dorjee, 2019).

What is going on here?

In my experience, many clients have a hard time being compassionate towards themselves, and as a result may feel uncomfortable engaging in self-compassion exercises, especially if they do not believe they are worthy of such compassion.

ACTION STEP

What should we do if one of our clients is being deeply affected by depression or rumination, and wants to seek professional mental help?

Refer them to a trained mindfulness-based cognitive-behavioral therapist (MBCT). According to researchers, mindfulness-based cognitive therapy (MBCT) is based on MBSR with a cognitive approach. This type of cognitive-behavioral therapy (CBT) was developed as a relapse prevention for people with chronic depression, and has been found to reduce the risk of depression relapse by half.

Studies also suggest that both MBCT and CBT are effective ways to enhance mindfulness and self-compassion and ease depression, anxiety, stress, and rumination in clients with anxiety, depression, and/or stress difficulties.

Moreover, researchers have found that people differ in their responses to meditation practices, and that MBCT may be more effective at enhancing mindfulness in people who experience excessive rumination (Frostadottir & Dorjee, 2019).

Therefore, I invite you to find a trained mental health professional in your area who utilizes MBCT so you can refer your clients to them, if needed.

You can find mindfulness-based cognitive-behavioral therapists here: https://www.psychologytoday.com/us/therapists/mindfulness-based-mbct

What is acceptance?

Acceptance is the act of recognizing and allowing one's current reality. As I stated earlier, mindfulness involves a nonjudgmental acceptance, and is designed to help people more effectively cope with stressful situations.

But doesn't mindfulness just focus on breathing and clearing your mind? What is so special about acceptance?

If our clients need to reduce the negative effects of stressors in their life, telling them to sit still and breathe while they hate every minute of the experience will be counterproductive. In the article, "Psychological

Mechanisms Driving Stress Resilience in Mindfulness Training: A Randomized Controlled Trial" researchers found that "acceptance skills training may be a necessary active ingredient … in stress-reduction interventions" (Chin et al., 2019).

What is acceptance and why is it so important?

First, acceptance is not the same thing as being weak or giving up. Rather, it is closer to "seeing things more clearly." In fact, Chin et al. state that acceptance is an emotion regulation skill that fosters non-reactivity, an openness to be present during experiences. Thus, the removal of acceptance skills training could reduce or eliminate the stress-buffering benefits of mindfulness interventions (2019). Clients with trauma histories tend to suffer from the effects of chronic toxic stress, so acceptance is an important and beneficial part of the practice.

ACTION STEP

How do we use this insight in our coaching?

Perhaps we can invite our clients to adopt "a gentle and accepting attitude towards sensory experiences and the fact that human minds wander." We might ask our clients if they would like to "invite in experiences with curiosity and interest, and to adopt a non-judgmental and accepting attitude towards their monitored experiences regardless of whether they are positive, negative, or neutral?" (Chin et al., 2019)?

ACTION STEP

What does acceptance look like?

I practice acceptance through self-compassion. According to Dr. Kristen Neff, self-compassion begins with a compassionate (mindful) awareness of one's suffering, and then encourages the suffering individual to repeat four statements to themself:

- "This is a moment of suffering." (This gently acknowledges pain without judging or immediately trying to "fix it," which can create tension.).
- "Suffering is a part of life." (This reminds us that we are all in the same boat. In other words, we all suffer at some point, and we all want to be happy. You are not alone.).
- "How can I add compassion to this moment?" (Compassion can elicit beneficial changes in the brain and body.).
- "How can I give myself the kindness I need right now?" (Studies indicate that kindness is more motivating, and produces better functioning, than harsh criticism.) (Schiraldi, 2021).

PARADIGM SHIFT

What might not work?

What might not work - using mindfulness as a shortcut by saying "just be mindful" to someone in the throes of a stressful situation. Let's take a look at what is happening when we are under stress. Often, our bodies react to stressors by becoming either hyperaroused or hypoaroused.

Fight-or-flight response

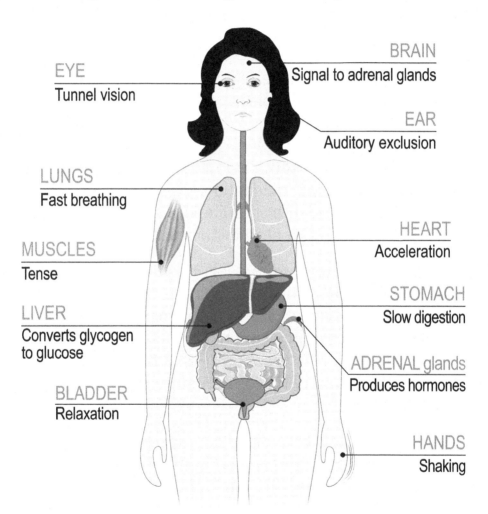

EYE
Tunnel vision

LUNGS
Fast breathing

MUSCLES
Tense

LIVER
Converts glycogen
to glucose

BLADDER
Relaxation

BRAIN
Signal to adrenal glands

EAR
Auditory exclusion

HEART
Acceleration

STOMACH
Slow digestion

ADRENAL glands
Produces hormones

HANDS
Shaking

Let's define hyperarousal and hypoarousal.

Hyperarousal occurs when our "fight-or flight" stress reaction is present. Symptoms may include sleep disturbances, inattention, anxiety, anger, defensiveness, restlessness, panic, and self-destructive behaviors.

Hypoarousal occurs when our "freeze," "fawn," or "tend and befriend" stress reaction is present. Symptoms may include excessive sleep, a feeling of emptiness or emotional numbness, a lack of motivation, dissociation, brain fog, inattention, and/or poor decision-making skills. Interestingly, some people confuse dissociation and hypoarousal with meditation goals and being a good meditator. The 'goal' of meditation is not to withdraw from life, numb out or stop thinking altogether.

Dissociation is not bad in itself; however, for some the main goal of dissociation is being a "people-pleaser," behaving in a specific way or performing certain acts in an effort to avoid conflict or ensure that the other person in the interaction is pleased (Perry & Winfrey, 2021). After a while, this behavior can start to have negative consequences.

Ironically, "Just be mindful!" appears to be the 21st-century version of telling someone who is upset to "just calm down." In the book, *Trauma Sensitive Mindfulness*, David Treleaven suggests to "consider again the potential implications of asking someone with dysregulated arousal to meditate. If they're hyperaroused, they may be facing intrusive imagery, traumatic sensations and disorganized cognitive processing. If they're hypoaroused, they may experience an absence of feeling, dissociation and disabled cognitive processing" (Treleaven, 2018).

Asking a client to 'Just be mindful' may appear to be dismissive of the client's legitimate distress and pain. So, if we are not discerning, the invitation to be mindful may be interpreted as dismissive of their trauma-based dread and shame (Treleaven, 2018).

Does that mean we should not recommend meditation at all?

Of course not! We can help people self-soothe their nervous system with grounding techniques that bring the feeling of safety and help regulate their nervous system. We can also teach them other skills that may be useful for them in stressful situations. We will learn more about these techniques later in the book.

Perfectionism - Will mindfulness still work if we are convinced we are "doing it wrong?"

Basic mindfulness interventions may not be useful for clients with maladaptive perfectionistic tendencies. Perfectionists may not get stress-reduction benefits from mindfulness practices that solely focus on breathing. Stress-related maladaptive perfectionism could potentially hinder the relaxation process (Azam et al., 2015).

What is maladaptive perfectionism?

Maladaptive perfectionism describes a continuous striving for unrealistic personal standards, an excessive concern over mistakes, and an attentional bias for failure. Excessive perfectionism is also linked to chronic stress, extreme worry, and high rumination levels (Azam et al., 2015).

In the article, "Heart Rate Variability is Enhanced in Controls but Not Maladaptive Perfectionists During Brief Mindfulness Meditation Following Stress-Induction: A Stratified-Randomized Trial," researchers found that perfectionists typically do not display a substantial heart rate variability (HRV) increase when exposed to brief mindfulness training. HRV is an indicator of well-being, with a lack of HRV serving as a signal that the person may be experiencing stress.

When contrasted with the control response, the lack of HRV appears to increase in perfectionists during mindfulness meditation, which suggests a maladaptive response to what the participant would want to be a relaxing practice.

Mindfulness interventions often ask people to remain seated in a relaxed and upright position with their eyes closed. The randomized trial used a ten minute audio recording, featuring mindfulness instructions, emphasizing attention to breathing sensations, and reorienting these breathing sensations once there is an awareness of one's thoughts, emotions, bodily sensations, and/or any external stimuli.

Why does this happen?

Experiential avoidance. Coping with maladaptive perfectionism and excessive worry involves avoidance - the tendency to avoid paying attention to undesirable sensations, emotions, and thoughts. A mindfulness intervention that focused on reorienting to the breath caused some people to experience an extreme fear of making mistakes, and an attentional bias for failure (Azam et al., 2015).

Has a client, friend or colleague who seems to be a perfectionist ever told you that they just don't like meditation or that it's too difficult for them?

PARADIGM SHIFT

What might NOT work?

Focusing on only spiritual musings, daily affirmations, or good vibes!

Shouldn't we tell our clients to eliminate their negative thoughts, and just focus on daily positive affirmations?

Instructions to "think positively" are common in North America. Self-help books, television shows, and loved ones often advise people to think positively when faced with challenges or when unhappy. Yet, research suggests that for certain people, positive self-statements may be ineffective and detrimental. Researchers have found that if people are allowed to focus on contradictory thoughts, along with affirmative thoughts, they are more equipped to handle stressors than if they did not combine these two actions. This may be especially true for people who unsuccessfully struggle to avoid negative thoughts (Wood et al. 2009).

Wood also found that "among participants with low self-esteem, those who repeated a positive self-statement ("I'm a lovable person") or who focused on how that statement was true felt worse than those who did not repeat the statement or who focused on how it was both true and not true" (2009).

This fantastic insight may help our clients who want the benefit of affirmations, but are unsure if they will work for them. Cohen and Sherman found that "self-affirmations can have lasting benefits when they involve a cycle of adaptive potential, a positive feedback loop between the self-systems, and a social system that gradually generates adaptive outcomes" (2014).

Could our clients use positive affirmations, while accepting (without judgment) that these statements may be both true and untrue?

ACTION STEP

How can we address our inner critic?

Dr. Kristin Neff, author, professor, and self-compassion researcher, teaches that our "inner critics" are simply trying to *help us*. As a result, she recommends that you refrain from beating yourself up for beating yourself up in an attempt to stop beating yourself up. Instead, take a step back, and give your inner critic some slack. In an ineffective, counterproductive way, your inner critic is actually trying to keep you safe (n.d.).

Are the critical voices in our heads harmless?

No, they are not! Neff explains that our stress levels rise as our amygdala activates our sympathetic nervous system (so we can deal with threats and danger) and floods our system with adrenaline and cortisol. This type of chronic stress can eventually lead to anxiety and depression, undermining our physical and emotional well-being (n.d.).

What does Neff recommend doing after we realize how our inner critics are holding a ruminative dialogue?

The next time you find yourself in the throes of harsh self-criticism, rather than beating yourself up for beating yourself up, thank your inner critic for its efforts, then try to give yourself some compassion instead (Neff, n.d.).

Later in the book, we will learn more about compassion meditation.

Why is understanding our inner critic so important?

Because self-criticism is detrimental to our self-care. Self-criticism activates our threat defense systems. In other words, when we sense danger, the amygdala sends signals that increase our blood pressure, adrenaline, and cortisol (Germer & Neff, 2019).

What type of mindfulness is best for a self-critic?

According to Germer and Neff, mindfulness practitioners who are self-critical may find it hard to consistently practice mindfulness until they are able to engage their inner critics. Therefore, self-critical people may benefit from practicing self-compassion *before* taking mindfulness training (2019).

The Bottom Line: ACEs can cause a dysregulated or uncontrolled stress response that involves a very high reactivity to stress, or a very low or blunted reactivity to stress.

Behaviors like being self-critical, perfectionistic, and/ or ruminating can boost stress hormones in the body. Mindfulness, acceptance, and self-compassion may help; however, the answer is more nuanced than just telling someone to go meditate and think good thoughts. Some interventions may be more effective than others in this population.

Let's finish the chapter with a moment of mindfulness.

The Fist Exercise

- First, make a fist, and imagine that your fist is balled up to protect you after a traumatic event.
- Next, use your other hand to try to pry your fist open.
- Then, release your fist.
- Take a moment to think about how that felt in your fist and in your entire body.
- Now, make a fist again.
- Instead of trying to pry it open, hold your other hand underneath it (supporting your closed fist with curiosity, kindness, and an understanding that it is protecting you after a traumatic event with a hand there to support you).
- Release your fist.
- Take a moment to think about how that felt in your fist and in your entire body.

Did you notice if your fist is a little tighter in one situation than the other? What bodily sensations did you notice during each of these situations?

We can either try to pry our clients open or understand and support them.

Based on this exercise, which approach would work better with your clients?

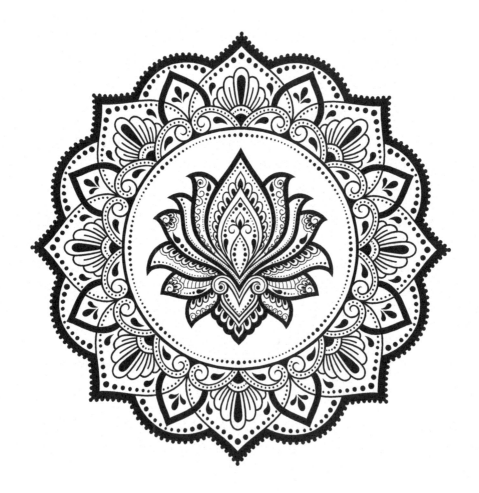

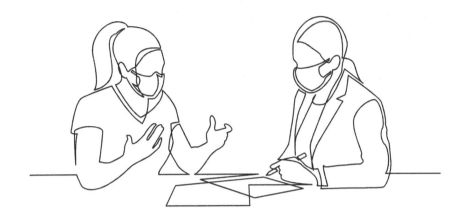

CHAPTER 4

KEEPING OURSELVES SAFE: WHAT IS SECONDARY TRAUMA?

Negative self-talk? Rumination? Emotional numbness? Wait! That sounds like me!

If this sounds like you too, let's look at secondary trauma.

What is secondary trauma? It is a type of trauma that occurs when a person is repeatedly exposed to other people's traumatic experiences.

In the article, "Secondary Trauma: Emotional Safety in Sensitive Research," Williamson et al. state secondary trauma (ST) is indirect exposure to traumatic events. The term is often used interchangeably with "vicarious trauma," "burnout," and "compassion fatigue" to convey ideas about the transference, or rippling effects, of trauma from the original incident and the original victim-survivor (2020).

What does secondary trauma feel like and when should we be concerned about it?

Well, we can ask ourselves a few questions:

- Can we "be present" for our clients when they share their traumatic stories?
- Instead of creating a safe space, are we numbing our own pain, or using our own defense mechanisms during client interactions?
- Do we feel detached from or hopeless about our work?

Whether or not we feel these symptoms, it is always a good idea to practice self-care.

How can we limit the impact of secondary trauma and still care for ourselves?

Limiting Exposure to Traumatic Work Experiences

A recent study on secondary trauma calming techniques found that it is beneficial to take breaks at work, refrain from work late at night, prevent your job from bleeding into your personal life, and limit your exposure to graphic images and sounds (Baker et al., 2020).

What does this look like in my life? My husband enjoys watching bloody psychological thrillers and horror movies, but I find the content to be too upsetting, so I leave the room when they are on. I read news online so I can choose which stories are most informative instead of watching news on TV, which can be too graphic and sensational. I also make sure I have a buffer in between when I consume potentially upsetting content and my bedtime.

Meditation, Exercise and Sleep

What else can we do?

Other recommended self-care practices include "meditation and mindfulness, regular exercise, adequate sleep" and researchers found that "some respondents explained that meditation helped center them, cleared their minds, and reduced anxiety. Respondents also said that sleep and exercise helped increase energy levels" (Baker et al., 2020).

It is important to note that according to Baker et al., "on meditation in particular, some respondents remarked that they had not found it useful, as it stressed them out or they could not stop their mind from wandering." The researchers did not inquire about how meditation was initially learned (2020). If you feel that meditation stresses you out or are frustrated that your mind does not completely stop wandering, alternative meditation practices may work better for you. We covered some potential reasons why meditation is stressful for some people in the previous chapter.

Cultivate Self-Compassion and Social Support

Self-compassion is not being self-indulgent, self-coddling, or spoiled. Practicing self-compassion does not mean that you will lose your motivation and drive to accomplish your goals.

According to the article, "An Investigation Into Compassion Fatigue and Self-Compassion in Acute Medical Care Hospital Nurses: A Mixed Methods Study," self-compassion involves three main components:

- "Self-kindness" or self-soothing and self-caring
- "Common humanity," or recognizing that no one is perfect, and we all make mistakes
- "Mindfulness" or being aware or "present" in the moment

Upton advises that instead of reacting to an unpleasant situation with self-criticism and harshness, clients could choose to be compassionate toward themselves. Why? Because a person who practices self-compassion puts suffering into perspective, and acknowledges and accepts that they are not alone in this suffering. In other words, this person exhibits kindness and compassion not just toward other people, but also toward themselves (Upton, 2018).

Social support is important, especially if we work alone in our practices. According to psychiatrist Bessel Van der Kolk, social support is not the same as being in the presence of others. The issue is reciprocity - being truly heard and seen by the people around us, and/or feeling that we are in someone else's mind and heart. "For our physiology to calm down, heal and grow we need a visceral feeling of safety" (2014).

Fortunately, we can find social support in person or in online groups. Social support from our peers can ultimately help us feel like we are seen and heard.

ACTION STEP

Try these self-compassion meditation tips from Dr. Kristin Neff: https://self-compassion.org/guided-self-compassion-meditations-mp3-2/

ACTION STEP

Thinking of all we have learned about trauma and toxic stress, could it be that some of our "common sense" beliefs about how people should behave are preventing us from seeing these behaviors as trauma responses?

How resilient are you? Answer these resilience survey questions from Origins Training and Counseling: https://originstraining.org/aces/resilience-survey/

Answers like "I am loveable," "I can ask for help," and/or "I can say no" can provide us with important insights into our resiliencies, especially when they involve relationships, internal beliefs, initiatives, and/or self-control (Resilience Survey, n.d.)

What really pushes our buttons?

In some cases, helping others exposes our own emotional triggers.

What are your emotional triggers?

Anger and Frustration Triggers

- People who intentionally hurt others (i.e., bullies).
- People who do not try or who *always* have an excuse (i.e., lazy).
- People who do not listen to others or care what others have to say (i.e., apathetic).
- People who are disrespectful (i.e., bad attitude).

- People who make excuses or blame others for their actions (i.e., irresponsible).
- People who are arrogant, prejudiced, or who frequently exclude others (i.e., rude).
- People who lack manners or common courtesy (i.e., spoiled).
- People who mock or criticize others (i.e., negativity).

Sadness and Disappointment Triggers

- When people do not live up to my expectations
- A belief that people are not as loving or caring as they should be
- Observing people who are hungry or "down on their luck"
- Watching someone try hard, but constantly fail
- Stories about tragedies or about people who have difficult lives
- People who give up
- Rejection

These triggers come from the Community Resilience Initiative Trauma Informed Certification Course 1.

I find myself affected by some of these triggers, especially when I have been experiencing stressful situations. If I see myself start to react to my own judgment of a situation, I need to be aware of my own dysregulation instead of blaming it on the situation or the person I am supposed to be helping. If we find ourselves overreacting to the stories we are telling ourselves, like 'people who have an excuse are just lazy,' we can end up retraumatizing our clients. We'll learn more about retraumatization in the next chapter.

Bottom Line: If we help traumatized individuals, even if we consider our work a 'calling,' we are still experiencing secondary trauma. We can have the best of intentions and still find ourselves triggered by judgemental thoughts. Feeling 'burned out' is normal and does not mean we are not meant for the work we love. We are invited to practice self-compassion and other self-care activities to help reduce the effects of secondary trauma.

Let's finish this chapter with a moment of mindfulness.

4-7-8 Breathing Exercise

Let's try four rounds of four-, seven-, and eight-count breathing exercises

1. Inhale (breathe in) for four counts.
2. Hold your breath for seven counts.
3. Exhale (breathe out) for eight counts.
4. Repeat this exercise three more times.

How did you feel after completing this short breathing exercise?

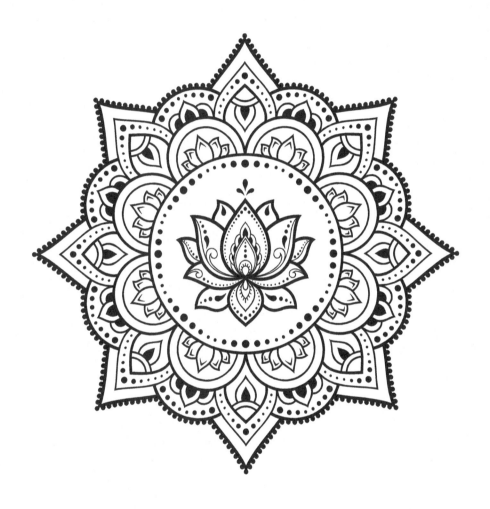

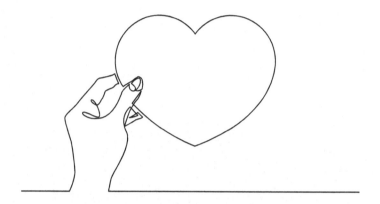

CHAPTER 5

KEEPING OUR CLIENTS SAFE: WHAT IS RE-TRAUMATIZATION?

How can we avoid re-traumatizing our clients and what steps can we take to provide "trauma-aware services?"

What is re-traumatization?

According to the handout, "Tips for Survivors of a Disaster or other Traumatic Event: Coping with Re-traumatization" published by the Substance Abuse and Mental Health Services Administration, some people's traumatic stress reactions to a new event may feel like re-experiencing an earlier event or events all over again.

This is known as re-traumatization. Re-traumatization is essentially reliving stress reactions experienced as a result of a traumatic event when faced with new, similar incidents (n.d.).

Here are some risk factors for re-traumatization:

- Having a high frequency of life traumas, such as chronic abuse or neglect
- Being emotionally "disconnected" from others or not feeling love and support from family members, peers, colleagues, friends, and/or other loved ones
- Living or working in unsafe situations
- Using unhealthy coping styles, such as avoidance or denial, and/or mismanaging stress (e.g., misusing alcohol, prescription medication, and/or illegal substances)
- Lacking economic and/or social support, or lacking proper access to healthcare services (Tips for Survivors of a Disaster, n.d.).

Healthcare providers can re-traumatize clients by:

- Treating clients like they are just numbers
- Attaching labels to clients, and/or using stigmatizing terms like "smoker" or "addict"
- Not providing clients with the power to make choices in their own treatment
- Not truly 'seeing' or 'listening' to clients

Unfortunately, many healthcare systems are set up to encourage re-traumatization. As a result, some clients have a distrust for us based on their previous experiences with other healthcare providers.

Giving Our Clients Control of Their Healthcare

Toxic stress can trigger changes in the reasoning and decision-making parts of the brain. Trauma occurs when there is a loss of control over personal safety, and some people with a history of trauma have trauma responses when they feel like they are re-experiencing a loss of control. Often, the trauma occurred at the hands of someone who was supposed to care for them.

How does this apply to us?

It is our job to help our clients. However, the act of helping exerts some level of control over the person we are trying to help.

What can different ways our client's handle control look like?

- Giving up all control (e.g., "Just tell me what to do!")
- Not wanting to give up any control (e.g., "Spare me the lecture!" or "No one tells me what to do!")

- Being unconvinced that we are here to collaborate with them (e.g., "I am only here because my doctor told me to come see you" or "Aren't you the one who is supposed to tell me all the answers?")

So, there really is an element of control in our roles as mind / body professionals, in that we provide our clients with advice, and lead them through practices. Our clients then react to our advice and instructions.

Keep in mind that our clients may be nervous at first. Thus, it is critical that we build trust with them. However, building trust by showing off what we know may be detrimental for some clients.

Two ways that we may be exacerbating our clients' hyperarousal states are:

- Overanalyzing the initial visit—too many questions may be overwhelming for some clients
- Rushing to tell the clients how to "fix" their problems *before* fully engaging with them

PARADIGM SHIFT

If the person we are helping has a trauma history, they may have a 'trauma response' to our action of helping because they are experiencing hyperarousal and/or perceive a loss of control. The 'trauma response' may happen even if we had the best intentions when we helped them and/or if the consequence of our assistance was beneficial to the person with a trauma history.

What our clients are experiencing is a loss of control, causing them to become defensive to our ways of helping. Our clients must feel safe, both intellectually and emotionally, to fully engage in behavior modification techniques. Also, understand that our clients' current behaviors are attempts to protect themselves from further trauma and cope with toxic stress.

ACTION STEP

What can we do to mitigate this?

Most mind / body professionals with behavioral modification training already practice many of these skills. We **ASK** and offer choices to our clients.

What does that look like?

It looks like the following:

- **ASKING** if the client is okay with accepting our assistance *before* diving in and "fixing" the problem.
- **ASKING** the client if they *want* our help.
- **RESPECTING** the answer, especially if it is "no." Keep in mind that the client may be in the precontemplation stage. Therefore, it is important to treat them as an expert in their life.

- If they agree, **ASK** how we can best help them instead of imposing our preferred way of helping on them. "When you're feeling like this, what helps you?"
- **INCORPORATING** the client's cultural experiences, knowledge, and learning processes into our coaching style. How can we support how our clients learn within their individual communities?
- **EXPLAINING** what we are going to do *before* helping.
- **ASKING** the client if what we are doing is helping them.
- **CHECKING** on the client's mental and physical health during the process.
- After the client has received our assistance, **ASKING** them if the help was beneficial. Do not forget to validate the client's feelings, thoughts, opinions, and experiences. Remember, our clients are the experts in their lives.
- **SHARING** ways the client could be self-sufficient in the future – but only after they **ASK** for our input. If so, we can use the strengths-based coaching model to collaborate in developing wellness strategies for our clients.

Bottom Line: Trauma occurs when there is a loss of control over personal safety. If we want to help our clients with their trauma histories while delivering services and resources to them in a trauma-informed manner, it is imperative that we understand the nature of trauma, and participate in trauma-informed care training.

The book *Trauma-Sensitive Mindfulness: Practices for Safe and Transformative Healing* by David Treleaven and Cheetahhouse.org are good resources for learning more about trauma and mindfulness.

Let's finish the chapter with a moment of mindfulness.

Sound Awareness Meditation

1. Sit quietly for six breaths and listen to the sounds surrounding you.

How did you feel after completing this exercise?

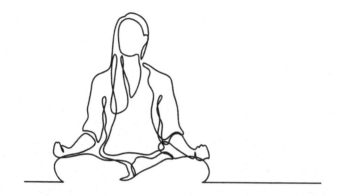

CHAPTER 6

CAN WE TRACK THE BENEFITS OF MINDFULNESS?

Why should we recommend mindfulness to our clients?

We learned earlier in the book that certain types of meditation are ***not*** recommended for people with low self-esteem, perfectionistic tendencies, and/or those who are critical of themselves. These clients may tell us, "I tried meditating before and it wasn't for me. I can't sit still for that long."

Can we track the benefits of mindfulness so we demonstrate to our clients that it is worth learning?

This is a tricky question, because many people believe that mindfulness should:

- Help stop their intrusive thoughts
- Make their problems go away
- Help them become calm and happy *all* the time

It is important to be open to our clients about why we are suggesting mindfulness interventions to them. Many of the benefits of mindfulness are overlooked, especially when people focus on mindfulness as a shortcut to solving *all* problems.

Let's look at the factors of mindfulness that may positively affect clients who are grappling with ACEs.

Mindfulness may help our clients cope with the stressors in their lives. ACEs can worsen adult mental health issues, in part because of changes in the structure and function of the body's stress-response systems. How? McKeen et al., state that "mindfulness is a cognitive resource that provides individuals with the tools necessary to deal with stress in a productive and healthy manner" (McKeen et al., 2021).

What are these tools? Mindfulness practice can improve our ability to:

- Observe the world around us
- Describe our feelings, beliefs, and opinions in detail

- Be self-aware
- Be nonjudgmental of our inner experiences
- Be nonreactive to our inner experiences

Why are these aspects of mindfulness important?

McKeen et al. state that negative cognitions, linked to ACEs, could harm a person's ability to effectively describe their feelings and be fully aware of the present moment, which could also contribute to symptoms of depression (2021).

Let's take a moment to really let this sink in.

Would our clients' perceptions of life improve if they could more effectively observe the world around them, describe their feelings, beliefs, and opinions in-depth, be more self-aware, and be nonjudgmental and nonreactive to their inner experiences?

Multiple studies have found that a decline in mindfulness may be linked to ACEs, and may contribute to the development of depression. ACEs may also hinder an individual's ability to develop healthy and productive coping mechanisms and mental resources that can help deal with life stressors. The researchers also found that the self-awareness element of mindfulness can moderate the relationship between ACEs and depression, such that a high level of self-awareness could serve as a protective factor against depression even as the number of ACEs increases (McKeen et al., 2021).

Mindfulness may also be beneficial for clients who want to reduce their substance use. In the article, "Mindfulness as a Mediator of the Association Between Adverse Childhood Experiences and Alcohol Use and Consequences," Brett et al. state that targeted alcohol treatment efforts that include mindfulness skills may be especially beneficial for people who have experienced early-life adversities (2018). McKeen et al. also found that nonjudgement and acting with self-awareness are the best protective factors in the relationship between ACEs, heavy alcohol use, and the related consequences (2021).

Keep in mind that mindfulness and stress reduction practices that we model should **not** be used as a substitute for professional behavioral health treatment. If our clients have questions and want to learn more about how mindfulness can help these issues, great! We can provide them with a referral for a local behavioral health treatment provider.

You can find behavioral health treatment providers here: https://findtreatment.samhsa.gov/

How can our clients use the five aspects of mindfulness to track their mindfulness journeys?

One way is to complete the Five Facets Mindfulness Questionnaire. You can find the questionnaire at https://ogg.osu.edu/media/documents/MB%20Stream/FFMQ.pdf

Bottom Line: Brief mindfulness interventions will **not** solve systemic problems, like being overworked and underpaid. These interventions may, however, offer opportunities to develop tools and coping mechanisms that help our clients embrace self-acceptance and a greater self-awareness. Returning to the object of focus (without judgment) when intrusive thoughts occur, during meditation is a good way for clients to practice these skills. Having thoughts during meditation is NOT a sign that our clients are bad at meditating.

PARADIGM SHIFT

The goal of meditation is not to just have positive thoughts and feelings. We should instead celebrate changes in our ability to notice our feelings, describe our feelings, watch our feelings without judgment or criticism, and consciously respond instead of react to our feelings.

Let's finish the chapter with a moment of mindfulness.

The Happiness Exercise

Let's send good wishes to someone that we love for the length of six breaths.

Silently say the following phrases:

- "May you be happy."
- "May you be healthy."
- "May you have ease of being."

How did you feel after completing this short compassion exercise?

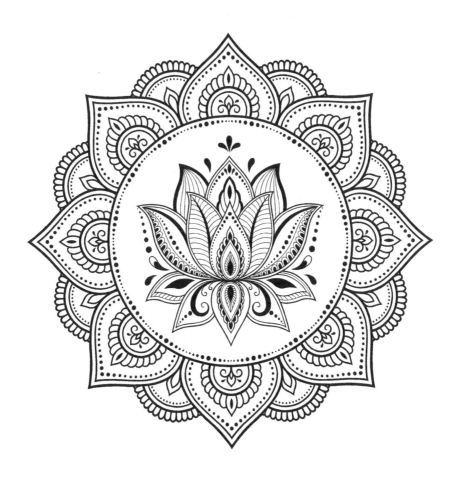

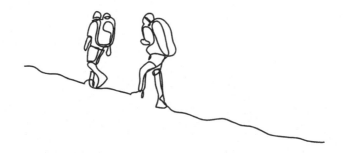

CHAPTER 7

MINDFUL INTERVENTIONS

How can we make a positive difference in our clients' lives?

We can go above and beyond just reducing unwanted symptoms and instead focus on improving their health – a concept referred to as "salutogenesis."

What is salutogenesis?

According to UCSD professor Robert K. Naviaux, the word "salutogenesis," coined by the Israeli-American medical sociologist Aaron Antonovsky, is used to describe the lifestyle choices and coping skills associated with the production and preservation of one's health, despite one's sociologic, economic, and/ or environmental hardships (Naviaux, 2021).

Why is salutogenesis important?

Mastering resilience practices can help reduce the negative effects of stressors on the body. Keep in mind that when something challenging occurs, the body perceives this as a stressor.

Common ways that we experience stressors include:

- Too much stress (good or bad) for a person's current resources
- Stress that is potentially dangerous to a person's health and well-being

When resilience practices provide us with additional resources, we are more equipped to handle stressors in our environment.

What does being more equipped to handle stressors mean?

It means that we do not automatically trigger a stress response in our bodies as quickly, which means we produce fewer stress-related hormones.

The State of California has created an important resource for children and adults with ACEs titled 'Roadmap for Resilience: The California Surgeon General's Report on Adverse Childhood Experiences, Toxic Stress, and Health.' Lead author Dr. Devika Bhushan serves as

California's acting surgeon general. The document is a "blueprint" for how communities, states, and nations can identify and effectively address ACEs. The researchers view toxic stress as a "root cause to some of the most harmful, persistent, and expensive societal and health challenges facing our world today" (California Surgeon General's Report, 2020).

The "Roadmap for Resilience" offers an integrative approach to ACEs and toxic stress in the following areas:

- Healthy relationships
- Quality sleep
- Balanced nutrition
- Regular physical activity
- Mindfulness
- Access to nature
- Behavioral and mental health care (Bhushan et al., 2020)

IMPORTANT: The general consensus is that *prevention,* during childhood, is far more effective than *interventions*, as an adult. Thus, it is also important to work towards preventing ACEs in the next generation.

PARADIGM CHANGE

"I'll sleep when I die."

"I'm too busy for self-care."

There is nothing surprising in the self-care practices listed in the Roadmap for Resilience. Just because we know something will be good for us does not mean we actually put it into practice. Resilience skills should not be tucked away until we experience a crisis. These positive coping skills are most beneficial when they become adaptive behaviors *before* they are needed to cope with stressful situations.

PARADIGM CHANGE

Self-care is about equity – not self-coddling.

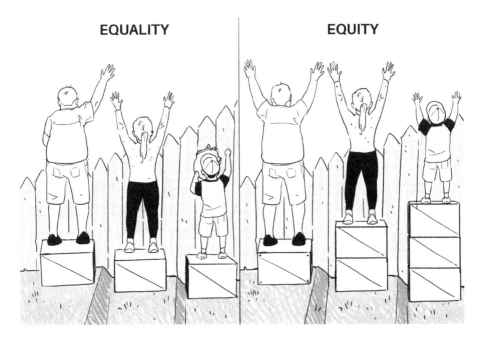

EQUALITY   EQUITY

Good self-care involves equity. Not all people need the same level of self-care. For example, if we have been affected by ACEs or have a chronic illness, we may need more self-care. Just because someone's life looks perfect from the outside, it does not necessarily mean they do not need to practice self-care.

If being blocked by the fence represents being outside of one's "window of tolerance," it makes sense that not all people need the same level of self-care. However, providing each person with the self-care they need helps them look over the fence (e.g., feeling the stability of being inside of one's window of tolerance).

Later in the book, we will learn more about windows of tolerance.

Lived Experiences

I would like to discuss the concept of sharing our lived experiences with our clients. Peer support is becoming a well respected part of healthcare. Many researchers have emphasized the importance of incorporating peer support into the healthcare system to instill hope; improve engagement, quality of life, self-confidence, and integrity; and reduce the burden on the healthcare system (Shalaby & Agyapong, 2020).

As a peer with our clients and in our communities, we can share our lived experience in trying the stress reduction strategies detailed later in the chapter. I invite you to not only think about your lived experiences, but also document your findings.

- What was easy?
- What was difficult?
- What improved your quality of life when you added it to your self-care routine?

Later in the chapter, we will focus on the strategies I listed above:

- Healthy relationships
- Good sleep quality
- Balanced nutrition
- Regular physical activity
- Mindfulness practices
- Time spent in nature and access to nature
- Behavioral and mental health care

But first, let's learn more about resilience.

What is Resilience?

Resilience is the ability to adapt to challenging circumstances and find a way to thrive, despite experiencing trauma. Ortiz & Sibinga describe resilience as successfully coping with adversity after experiencing trauma (2017). It is important to note, however, that these resilience skills will not provide us with carefree lives.

Instead, they may help us more effectively respond to the difficulties we encounter in life.

Healthy Relationships

As a lymphedema therapist, I have seen firsthand that having support and experiencing a sense of belonging and community is vital to the long-term health of people with chronic illnesses. Daily self-care is mandatory for maintaining a high quality of life when one struggles with lymphatic disorders like lymphedema and lipedema. Self-care is more difficult without a strong support system.

Do your clients enjoy getting support from loved ones, and do they feel like they are members of a community?

According to Bhushan et al., the following questions may be used to gauge the level of perceived social support and integration:

- Do you feel like you have someone, who understands and believes in you, and who you can talk to when you become upset?"
- Is there someone who can provide you with emotional, financial, and material support? If so, who?
- Do you feel like you belong to a group or community? (California Surgeon General's Report, 2020).

Why is social support important?

Researchers suggest that relationships can ease stress and reduce or eliminate the negative health impacts of ACEs (California Surgeon General's Report, 2020).

How can we explore resilience with our clients?

German researchers have used the Brief Resilience Coping Scale (BRCS) to explore the "effects of childhood adversities and resilience on distress and somatic symptoms" in German adults.

The BRCS instructs participants to rate "how well each of four statements describe their behavior and actions:"

- "I look for creative ways to alter difficult situations."
- "Regardless of what happens to me, I believe I can control my reactions."
- "I believe I can grow in positive ways by dealing with difficult situations."
- "I actively look for ways to replace the losses I encounter in life" (Beutel, 2017).

Why are the answers important?

ACEs are associated with a heightened vulnerability in the area of low resilience coping mechanisms (e.g., in the areas of helplessness and low self-efficacy). Thus, people who report ACEs tend to have had less social support early in life, which could be considered a "social component of resilience." Thus, coping with the demands and challenges of life can be extremely difficult. Helplessness and low self-efficacy can negatively affect your ability to adaptively cope with conflicts. This, in turn, can lead to depression, anxiety, and somatic symptoms in adults who have experienced ACEs (Beutel, 2017).

Building Supportive Relationships and Creating Communities

Why are relationships important for our clients?

Dr. Perry shares that a person's history of relational health (i.e., connectedness to family, community, and culture) is more predictive of their mental health than their history of adversity. In other words, "connectedness has the ability to counterbalance adversity" (Perry & Winfrey, 2021).

One way to receive a feeling of "belonging" is to volunteer. Volunteering can help build supportive relationships. In fact, Philippus et al. found that volunteering can help improve a person's life satisfaction and encourage them to socialize and interact with people in the general population (2020).

In the book, *Drop the Skirt: How My Disability Became My Superpower,* Amy Rivera, who has primary lymphedema, shares how volunteering at a nursing home helped her realize that everyone has their own stories, and that everyone struggles with something at one point. Volunteering helped Rivera find her purpose. She found happiness in helping others (2021).

ACTION STEP

Clients can find volunteering opportunities in their community here: https://www.volunteermatch.org/

I am a member of my local Lions Club. Find more information at https://www.lionsclubs.org/

What are local volunteer resources you would like to share with your clients?

_____

_____

Practicing Gratitude

Practicing gratitude may help our clients build relationships. Lindberg states that people who are grateful are typically calmer and more peaceful. In other words, these individuals tend to be more positive, which can be attractive to other people. When a person has positive feelings and can relish good times with others, bonding occurs, which can lead to stronger relationships (2019).

What is gratitude?

Xiang et al. state that "gratitude can be defined as a complex subjective feeling including

- wonder,
- thankfulness,
- appreciation in one's life."

The researchers state that gratitude has positive effects, including:

- "subjective well-being,
- life satisfaction, and
- social relationships."

Gratitude may involve reflecting, motivating, and/or reinforcing social actions in both the "givers" and the "recipients." People with higher levels of gratitude may also obtain more social resources, especially social support from others. Researchers have found that grateful people typically have high levels of social support. Higher levels of social support can lead to higher levels of benign envy and lower levels of malicious envy (2018).

ACTION STEP

How can we practice gratitude?

- **Start a gratitude journal.** Write at least five sentences about something we are grateful for. Start with journaling several times a week and gradually increase the frequency until it becomes a daily practice.
- **Start with Three Things**. We can fit a quick gratitude practice into our daily routine. For instance, I can think of three things that I am grateful for while waiting for the water to warm up for my daily shower.

- **Sprinkle moments of gratitude into our social media feed.** I follow inspirational people on social media. TED speaker Andrew Bird offers gratitude meditations at @dreadfulbird on Instagram and TikTok.

Learn more about gratitude here: https://greatergood.berkeley.edu/topic/gratitude

What are gratitude practices you would like to share with your clients?

_____

_____

PARADIGM SHIFT

Understand that gratitude also has a dark side. In the white paper, "The Science of Gratitude," Allen suggests that people with disabilities, who rely on support for their care, often feel burdened by gratitude. Specifically, these individuals tend to feel "forced" to express gratitude to receive the support they need and end up feeling shame and frustration over the one-sided nature of their dependent relationships. Researchers have found that relationship problems can arise when gratitude becomes a type of "currency," in which one (or both) partners feel "underpaid" (2018).

Coach - Try It Yourself!

Have healthy relationships benefited your emotional well-being? If so, how?

Challenge yourself to keep a "gratitude journal" for a week.

What did you notice?

What are lived experiences you would like to share with your clients?

_____

_____

Quality Sleep

Sleep is an important part of maintaining one's health. "How much sleep are you getting each night?" is one of the questions I typically ask clients who are recovering from surgery.

Why is sleep so important?

According to Emory University researchers, people who sleep six hours or less each night have higher levels of three inflammatory markers (fibrinogen, IL-6 and C-reactive protein), as compared to individuals who sleep six hours or more each night (Poor Sleep Quality Increases Inflammation, 2010).

Many of my clients say that their sleep quality is not good during the post-surgery recovery process. It's worth it to ask more questions to pinpoint why - is it pain, discomfort from a new sleeping position, temperature, or another factor?

What are other common causes of insomnia?

A sleep hygiene study suggests that drinking alcohol, smoking near bedtime, and/or taking naps during the day can trigger or worsen insomnia (Jefferson et al, 2005).

ACTION STEP

Should we discuss sleep quality with our clients?

According to Bhushan et al., interrupted sleep or insomnia is one of the most common and nonspecific outcomes of childhood adversity.

The researchers recommend focusing on four key elements:

- How satisfied clients are with their sleep quality.
- How restored and rested clients feel upon waking up in the morning.
- How hard it is for them to fall asleep each night.
- How hard it is to stay asleep or fall back to sleep once awakened (California Surgeon General's Report, 2020).

You can find the National Institutes of Health's "Guide to Healthy Sleep" here: https://www.nhlbi.nih.gov/files/docs/public/sleep/healthy_sleep.pdf

ACTION STEP

Here are some tips on how to get a good night's sleep:

- **Banish blue light**. Consider getting a special light bulb for your lamp that eliminates blue light. The subdued amber glow could also help relax you before bed.

- **Use electronics wisely before bed**. I try not to look at my electronics (e.g., smartphone, laptop, desktop computer, television, tablets, etc.) for at least 30 minutes before my bedtime. However, I do use electronics to listen to soothing music or guided meditations before bed.

- **Develop a consistent sleep schedule**. I set an alarm for 30 minutes before my bedtime, so I can start prepping for bed. When I break my routine, I end up staying up hours after my bedtime. Then, when I awaken the next morning, I usually feel awful. So I make a habit of going to bed and waking up at the same time each day – even on the weekends.

- **Take a warm bath or shower**. If I feel too "energized" late in the evening, I might take a warm bath or shower to relax.

- **Read before bed**. Reading a few pages before bed helps my husband transition from daytime activities to sleep.

- **Soothe a restless mind with guided meditation.** I sometimes like to listen to sleep meditations on my smartphone until I fall asleep. Insight Timer is one of several free apps that offer a wide selection of meditations. I listen with earphones, so I do not bother my husband. Yoga nidra, body scan, and mantra meditation practices may help clients fall asleep faster. My father used to fall asleep to recordings of old radio programs from his youth. Encourage your clients to get creative and find stress-management techniques that work for them.

Yoga Nidra and Non-Sleep Deep Rest

Andrew Huberman, neuroscientist and professor in the Department of Neurobiology at the Stanford University School of Medicine, coined the term "non-sleep deep rest" (NSDR). Practices like yoga nidra (a stress-management technique) may help clients enter deeper states of rest, fall asleep more quickly, and reduce stress.

If you awaken in the middle of the night (which can be a normal occurrence once or twice a night), consider listening to a NSDR recording to help you fall back asleep. Huberman suggests that you search for 'NSDR' or 'yoga nidra' in YouTube and find a version that appeals to you (Huberman, 2021).

What is yoga nidra?

Yoga nidra is not the type of yoga that involves movement, poses, or working up a sweat. Yoga nidra involves entering into a "hypnogogic state." Researchers suggest that this type of yoga not only improves sleep, but it also encourages learning and self-control (Sharpe et al., 2021).

How does yoga nidra work?

According to Vaishnav, yoga nidra is an ancient Indian method that helps individuals enter into positive states of deep physical, mental, and emotional relaxation. This practice triggers simultaneous relaxation and detachment, leading to self-awareness and the release of stress. Thus, the goal of yoga nidra is to increase a person's ability to focus and improve health and well-being.

Researchers found that out of thirty-six children aged thirteen to fifteen who received yoga nidra sessions thirty minutes a day, three days a week, for one month, over half of the children experienced better focus in the classroom. The researchers also measured the students before and after the study with the Psychological General Well-Being Index (PGWBI) and found a significant difference in the PGWBI short subscale items that measure anxiety, vitality, depressed mood, self-control, positive well-being, and vitality (Vaishnav et al., 2018).

Yoga nidra may also be effective for anxiety issues that stem from a chronic illness. A study found that people aged eighteen to forty-five with menstrual problems/irregularities for longer than six months, who practice yoga nidra for at least thirty-five minutes, five days a week, for six months, may experience an improvement in their mild-to-moderate anxiety and depression symptoms. There does not appear to be significant improvement in people with severe anxiety or depression symptoms (Rani et al., 2012).

What tips on getting better sleep would you like to share with your clients?

Coach - Try It Yourself!

What sleep hygiene practices have made the most difference in your sleep habits? Which ones do you want to try? Can you challenge yourself to not use electronics for an hour before bed for at least a week?

What did you notice?

What are lived experiences you would like to share with your clients?

Balanced Nutrition

Is nutrition important for reducing the effects of toxic stress on the body? Stress is just all in our mind, right?

According to The Roadmap for Resilience, ACEs and toxic stress have been linked to insulin resistance, diabetes, and eating disorders (California Surgeon General's Report, 2020). Stress and nutrition can affect each other. More specifically, eating too little can activate your body's stress response (e.g., feeling "hangry" and irritable), and stressors can affect your metabolism and how well your body digests food.

Are our clients "stuck in a rut," making the same meals over and over?

Here is an informative handout listing the many options available in each category of foods. This could be a good resource for someone interested in trying new foods and recipes. https://www.dietaryguidelines. gov/sites/default/files/2021-11/DGA_2020-2025_ CustomizingTheDietaryGuidelinesFramework.pdf

Specific questions about nutrition and requests for customized eating plans can be referred to a Health at Every Size professional. Find one here: https://asdah. org/

What are lived experiences you would like to share with your clients?

_____

_____

PARADIGM SHIFT

Judging a person based on their weight is not only harmful, but also inaccurate. According to Bhushan et al., implying that a person's dietary choices and weight gain are solely the result of a lack of willpower and/or poor personal choices is biologically inaccurate. A trauma-informed approach can remove this stigma and help decrease blame and shame (California Surgeon General's Report, 2020).

PARADIGM SHIFT

Does your client have access to quality, fresh foods?

According to the USDA, in 2020, approximately 11% (14 million) of U.S. households were "food insecure" at some point. Food insecurity is defined as being uncertain of having, or unable to acquire enough food to meet the basic needs of the family because of insufficient funds or resources to purchase food (Key Statistics & Graphics, n.d.). Food insecurity can be a significant roadblock to forming healthy nutritional habits.

ACTION STEP

- "Feeding America" has a list of local food banks that you can find here: https://www.feedingamerica.org/find-your-local-foodbank
- You can find food assistance for military and veteran families here: https://www.fns.usda.gov/military-and-veteran-families

What local resources would you like to share with your clients?

_____

_____

Regular Physical Activity

For many people, exercising feels like a punishment or something they have to force themselves to do. How can we help our clients reframe this viewpoint? One idea is to start with rhythm.

Dr. Perry states that rhythm is essential for a healthy body and a healthy mind.

Most people can probably think of a song or beat that gets them moving and brightens their mood. Some types of movement have rhythm as well. Walking, swimming, and dancing are rhythmic ways you can add physical activity into your daily routine.

Dr. Perry also believes everyone has a specific go-to remedy when they feel "out of sync," anxious, and/ or frustrated. The common element? Rhythm (Perry & Winfrey, 2021). Would our clients be interested in enjoying an activity that involves rhythm?

Physical Activity and Brain Activity

Prolonged stress can change our brains - but regular physical activity can change our brains, too - and it can be as simple as walking every day.

How does it work?

Our body's stress response can shrink the hippocampus, the part of the brain associated with learning and memory. McEwen found that while prevention is the most effective and economical way to address ACEs (e.g., stemming from a perceived threat or danger), "treatments after the problems with physical and mental health have developed are also necessary." McEwen states that regular physical activity is a top-notch therapy that can improve blood flow to your prefrontal and parietal cortex and enhance your executive functions. Moreover, regular physical activity (e.g., walking one hour a day for five days a week) can increase hippocampal volume in previously sedentary adults. Thus, researchers have concluded that "physically fit" individuals have larger hippocampal volumes than sedentary adults of the same age (2012).

Cotman et al. found that exercise may help people who are struggling with depression. The researchers suggest that aerobic or resistance training exercise (for two to four months) may help ease depression in both young and older individuals. The benefits of exercise are comparable to the benefits of taking antidepressants and (up to a point) greater improvements occur with higher levels of exercise (2007).

Exercise can also trigger changes in the hypothalamic–pituitary–adrenal axis, the part of the brain that regulates the stress response and alters the dorsal raphe serotonin neurons, which are linked to "learned helplessness behaviors" (Cotman et al., 2007). What does this mean for our clients? Starting a habit of regular physical activity may help our clients whose learned helplessness behaviors are preventing them from making positive changes in their lives.

Exercise and "Learned Helplessness"

What is "learned helplessness?"

Learned helplessness, a phrase coined in 1967 by Dr. Martin Seligman and Dr. Steven Maier, is described as a person's behavior when they stop trying to "fix" or improve things after long-term exposure to uncontrollable situations.

Are our clients telling us that nothing they do matters, and/or are they exhibiting apathy and powerlessness?

According to Greenwood et al., depression and "learned helplessness" are behavioral consequences of being exposed to uncontrollable stressful events.

What happens in the brain?

Researchers state that serotonin (5-HT) neurons in the dorsal raphe nucleus (DRN) can promote learned helplessness (e.g., poor escape responding and expressing an exaggerated conditioned fear, and/or triggering an acute exposure to uncontrollable stress) (Greenwood et al., 2003).

What can help reduce the effects of uncontrollable stress?

Researchers found that, in an animal study, six weeks of voluntary freewheel running can reduce the behavioral effects of uncontrollable stress, supporting the hypothesis that, in animals, freewheel running can prevent learned helplessness (Greenwood et al., 2003).

Understand, however, that the exercise should be voluntary, not forced. Cotman et al. found that while forced exercise and voluntary exercise may be beneficial for learning and acquiring skills, voluntary exercise appears to produce the most reliable benefits. Although some studies show improvements after one week of exercise, most benefits are linked to long-term exercise (e.g., three to twelve weeks) (2007).

Let's look at some other types of exercise that could be beneficial for clients who are dealing with chronic stress.

Trauma-Informed Yoga

Is yoga a good form of exercise for clients with stress?

According to therapist Robyn Brickel, the nervous system of a trauma survivor is prepared for danger, and as such, can be in a constant state of hyperarousal or hypoarousal. Research suggests that yoga, meditation, and guided imagery can help to balance the nervous system, thereby bringing our clients down from a state of hyperarousal, and closer to a "window of tolerance" and "emotional regulation" (2017).

The practice should be guided by a trauma-informed expert. According to psychiatrist Bessel van der Kolk, about half of trauma survivors in his first yoga study stopped participating in yoga because they felt like it was too intense. Various yoga postures, especially those that involve the pelvis, can trigger panic attacks and/or sexual assault flashbacks and "intense physical sensations unleashed the demons from the past that had been so carefully kept in check by numbing and inattention" (2014).

PARADIGM SHIFT

Yoga may not be beneficial for all people. In an article for *Glamour* magazine, Susi Wrenshaw, yoga instructor, states that practicing yoga regularly can quiet your mind, so you experience a sense of connectedness and peace, free from your perceptions and projections. This can be challenging for trauma survivors as quietness can quickly overwhelm them and trigger dissociation or make them feel overwhelmed.

What is the goal of trauma-informed yoga?

According to Wrenshaw, trauma-informed yoga requires expertise in helping students recognize and remain in their "windows of tolerance," so they are neither over-activated (increasing the risk of flashbacks or panic attacks) or under-activated (triggering a shutdown in awareness) (Ward, 2021).

What are the components of trauma-informed yoga?

According to Wrenshaw, trauma-informed yoga involves grounding, self-awareness, stress management, and a fear response reduction. This type of yoga uses a variety of poses to ease stress and anxiety. A trauma-informed yoga teacher does not place their hands on the student. Rather, they develop clear boundaries by offering choices, and helping the student understand what is happening in their body and brain (Ward, 2021).

ACTION STEP

You can find a local yoga teacher here: https://www.yogaalliance.org/

What are local yoga resources you would like to share with your clients?

_____

_____

Walking the Labyrinth

What is a labyrinth?

A labyrinth is often confused for a maze, which has many dead ends and is meant to confuse the walker.

A true labyrinth is a simple geometric form where one path leads to the center. A labyrinth is often used in religious and health-related institutions for quiet walking and meditative processes. It can be a tool for reducing psychological and physical stress (Behman et al., 2018).

How can labyrinth walking benefit our clients?

In the article, "A Literature Review on the Physiological and Psychological Effects of Labyrinth Walking," Davis states that labyrinths are commonly used for therapy in diverse healthcare settings, such as cancer treatment centers, domestic violence shelters, healing gardens, nursing facilities, and major medical centers, like

Johns Hopkins Medical Center. People who walk the labyrinth report that doing so calms them, emotionally and spiritually, and helps them cope with their grief and make better decisions (2021).

A recent study indicates that some people experience immediate physiological arousal while walking the labyrinth, while others experience a heightened physiological awareness and relaxation during and/or after a labyrinth walk (Behman et al., 2018).

A Brazilian study found that one of the main objectives of a labyrinth is to improve attention and judgment-free present moment awareness, which is reached with walking the path of the labyrinth. Researchers suggest that walking a labyrinth can trigger contemplation, reflection, and transformation.

Data also indicate that walking a labyrinth is a form of psychoneuroimmunology that can be used in integrative patient care. Labyrinths can be used by nurses to help patients undergoing oncology treatments reach a contemplative and altered state of consciousness.

Researchers also found that the vast majority of people in one study reported emotional distress stemming from a feeling that the path was longer on the way out (Lizier et al., 2018). Because of this, clients should be told that it is OK to step out of a labyrinth when they reach the center or if they start to experience overwhelming emotional distress.

ACTION STEP

You can find a local labyrinth at labyrinthlocator.com.

Are there any local labyrinths you would like to share with your clients?

_____

_____

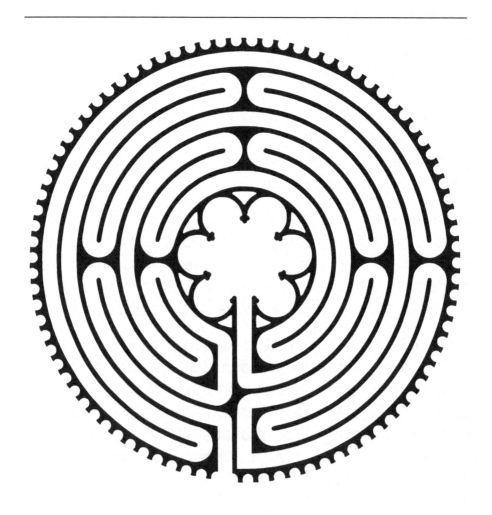

Qigong and Tai-Chi

Have you seen an individual or group of people in a park performing elegant, peaceful, and flowing movements? It could be Qigong or Tai Chi. These two practices involve coordinated body postures and movements, deep rhythmic breathing, meditation, and mental focus, based on traditional Chinese medicine theories (Yeung et al., 2018).

What are the benefits of these practices?

Qigong can be beneficial for people with depression and/or anxiety who are living with chronic health conditions. A recent study also found that Tai Chi can be beneficial for a wide range of measures of psychological well being, including depression, anxiety, stress, mood disturbances, self-esteem, and exercise efficacy (Yeung et al., 2018).

How might these practices benefit our clients?

Preliminary studies suggest that the slow movements and breathing in Qigong and Tai Chi may affect a person's nervous system and restore homeostasis (internal balance), reduce stress-related hypothalamus–pituitary–adrenal axis reactivity, and help regulate the autonomic nervous system functions toward parasympathetic dominance (Yeung et al., 2018).

ACTION STEP

Qigong and Tai-Chi can be practiced anywhere, at any time—without equipment.

You can learn more about Qigong and Tai Chi at https://www.nccih.nih.gov/health/tai-chi-and-qi-gong-in-depth

What are local Qigong and Tai Chi resources you would like to share with your clients? _____

_____

Coach—Try It Yourself!

If you do not have a regular yoga, labyrinth walking, Qigong and Tai Chi practice, challenge yourself to try 10-20 minutes of one new type of mindful movement a day for a week. Pay attention to timing the breath with your movements.

What did you notice?

What are lived experiences you would like to share with your clients?

_____

_____

Mindfulness

How can mindfulness help our clients?

Mindfulness has been proven to benefit individuals who have experienced trauma or ACEs by not only indirectly negating the body's acute response to trauma and stress, but also stopping, reducing, or preventing the possible underlying consequences of chronic exposure to them (e.g., psychiatric, metabolic and cardiovascular disease influenced by lifestyle choices, underlying biochemistry, and neurobiology) (Ortiz & Sibinga, 2017).

Mindfulness practices that embrace a non-judgemental approach could boost resilience in people who have experienced trauma, because it offers an alternative to the psychological dissociation that commonly occurs after trauma. Psychological dissociation can interfere with healthy processing and/or coping (Ortiz & Sibinga, 2017).

Characteristics of mindfulness include accepting one's thoughts, urges, beliefs, etc., without judgment, and being more self-aware—behaviors inversely associated with post-traumatic stress symptoms.

Why does this happen?

Mindfulness supports a nonjudgmental acceptance of painful and unpleasant thoughts and emotions and encourages decreased reactivity to these thoughts and emotions (Ortiz & Sibinga, 2017).

PARADIGM SHIFT

Acceptance is an important aspect of mindfulness. According to the article "Despite understanding the concept of mindfulness, people are applying it incorrectly, research shows" Dr. Igor Grossmann, social psychology professor at University of Waterloo, states that engaging with your stressors could provide some much-needed stress relief. Mindfulness includes two main components: awareness and acceptance. However, it is common to confuse acceptance with passiveness or avoidance (University of Waterloo, 2021). Understand that accepting something does not automatically mean avoiding it. Accepting is acknowledging its presence and allowing it to be a part of your experience in the present moment.

PARADIGM SHIFT

Mindfulness is **NOT** a way to force yourself to relax. Learning to be aware of and be with uncomfortable feelings are primary aspects of mindfulness. If you are not feeling peaceful after a short mindfulness session - that awareness too is mindfulness.

If a client just needs to relax and mindfulness meditation is not working, invite them to try the grounding exercises discussed later in the book.

Now, let's try a few mindfulness techniques

Let's start by practicing some simple breathwork, then explore different meditations you can introduce to clients. You are invited to assume a position that is alert, yet relaxed. You can close your eyes, if that feels right to you.

I have found that the majority of clients ask for a copy of the script or an audio version of the guided meditations I try with them, so I have given you those resources to pass along to your clients.

If your client has a habit of hyperventilating during deeper breathing exercises, have them try breathing through the nose, instead of through the mouth.

Box Breathing

Practice this exercise for a minute or two, if possible. If you become overwhelmed, turn to your grounding resources.

1. Inhale (breathe in) for two counts
2. Hold your breath for two counts
3. Exhale (breathe out) for two counts
4. Hold your breath for two counts
5. Repeat steps 1-4 for a minute or two
6. Open your eyes, move your fingers and toes, and/ or stretch

What did you notice?

4-7-8 Breathing

Try this exercise for two minutes. If you become overwhelmed, turn to your grounding resources.

1. Inhale (breathe in) for four counts
2. Hold your breath for seven counts
3. Exhale (breathe out) for eight counts
4. Repeat steps 1-3 for a minute or two
5. Open your eyes, move your fingers and toes, and stretch

What did you notice?

Self-Compassion Mindfulness

Living with a chronic illness can be hard. You are human, so it is only natural to feel frustrated about your condition. You are not alone.

Try this exercise for two minutes. If you become overwhelmed, turn to your grounding resources.

Follow these steps:

1. Say to yourself 'It is hard to experience this chronic illness'
2. Say to yourself 'This is part of being human, nothing wrong with feeling frustrated about your condition, I am not the only one'

3. Put a hand on your heart - say something kind to ourselves (What would you say to a friend struggling with a chronic illness or chronic stress?)

4. Ground yourself - feel your body against the furniture

5. Open your eyes, move your fingers and toes, and stretch

Loving-Kindness Meditation

Try this exercise for two minutes. If you become overwhelmed, turn to your resources.

First Minute

Think of a person or pet that is easy for you to love.

Silently repeat these phrases:

- *"May you be happy."*
- *"May you be healthy."*
- *"May you be safe."*
- *"May you have ease of being."*

Second Minute

Silently repeat these phrases:

- *"May I be happy."*
- *"May I be healthy."*
- *"May I be safe."*

- *"May I have ease of being."*

When you are finished, open your eyes, move your fingers and toes, and stretch.

Note: If the second part feels difficult or "fake," imagine a loved one saying these phrases to you instead.

Listed below are resources that your clients can use in-between visits. We can use our own voices to guide clients through these practices, or listen to prerecorded guided meditations with our clients, then send them the links, so they can listen to them in between sessions.

Encourage your clients to practice quick everyday mindfulness exercises like *"RAIN."* The RAIN exercise, created by Michele McDonald, is an easy-to-remember tool, designed to help with challenging emotions. It is also good for performing routine checks on your clients' daily experiences.

RAIN

- **Recognize** what is happening in and around us.
- **Allow** what is present to be.
- **Investigate** what is happening with kindness.
- **Nurture** and/or rest in a natural self-awareness.

Here is a resource you can share with your clients about this mindfulness meditation practice: https://www.tarabrach.com/rain/

STOP

The steps are:

1. **Stop** (Stop what we are doing)
2. **Take a Breath** (Pay attention as we take the next breath)
3. **Observe** (What are our current feelings and emotions? Are there any notable physical sensations in our body? We don't need to change or judge them, just observe them)
4. **Proceed** (Return to what we were doing).

Here is a resource that you can share with your clients about this practice: https://accelerate.uofuhealth.utah.edu/resilience/practice-s-t-o-p

Body Scan

Here is a quick three-minute body scan from Diana Winston: http://marc.ucla.edu/mpeg/Body-Scan-Meditation.mp3

Working with Difficult Emotions

Here is a more in-depth guided practice for challenging emotions from Kristin Neff: "Soften, Soothe and Allow:" https://self-compassion.org/wp-content/uploads/2020/08/softensootheallow_cleaned_01-cleanedbydan.mp3

More meditations from Kristin Neff:

- https://self-compassion.org/category/exercises/#guided-meditations
- https://cih.ucsd.edu/mindfulness/guided-audio-video

Free Smartphone Apps

- iBreathe
- iChill - Trauma Resource Institute
- Mindfulness Coach – Department of Veterans Affairs
- UCLA Mindful - Mindful Awareness Research Center

Local healthcare systems may provide clients with handouts on mindfulness.

- *Kaiser Permanente Mindfulness Meditation:* https://my.kp.org/pepperdine/wp-content/uploads/sites/840/2013/07/Mindfulness-flyer.pdf
- *Mindfulness for Those with COPD, Asthma, Lung Cancer, and Lung Transplantation:* https://www.thoracic.org/patients/patient-resources/resources/mindfulness.pdf
- *Mindfulness and Heart Health:* https://www.health.harvard.edu/heart-health/mindfulness-can-improve-heart-health
- *Take a Moment with Meditation from the American Cancer Society:* https://www.cancer.org/latest-news/take-a-moment-with-meditation.html
- *How to Lower Toxic Stress:* https://www.acesaware.org/wp-content/uploads/2020/01/Lower-Toxic-Stress-Handout-Adult-English.pdf
- *Share Mindfulness with Children:* https://www.acesaware.org/wp-content/uploads/2019/12/9-Using-Mindfulness-English.pdf

What are mindfulness meditation practices you would like to share with your clients?

_____

_____

Mindfulness and Art Therapy

For many people, the process of creating art is relaxing. Some people go further, using art therapy to purposely address trauma and reduce the impact of stress on their bodies. Art therapy is the methodical use of drawing, painting, collage, or sculpting to influence and express feelings, thoughts, and memories and involves "active performing and experiencing with art materials, by the visual and concrete character of the process as well as by the result of art making" (Schouten et al., 2014).

Mindfulness-based art therapy (MBAT) combines mindfulness practices with art therapy to promote health, wellness, and adaptive responses to stress. Recent studies suggest that intensive MBAT and other mindfulness-based interventions are beneficial for severe health conditions, such as cancer, heart disease, and anxiety (Beerse et al., 2020).

Playing with clay may also be an option for our clients. Research has found that clay carries natural therapeutic properties that could complement mindfulness, as the act of clay sculpting alone appears to trigger relaxation and a meditative state (Beerse et al., 2020).

The mandala is an ancient art form that is used in many cultures. In the article, "Empirical Study on the Healing Nature of Mandalas," people were asked to draw a large circle on paper, and fill in the circle with representations of their feelings or emotions, related to their traumas.

The individuals were then instructed to use symbols, patterns, designs, and colors (but no words) to describe how they were feeling. The drawing period lasted twenty minutes a day for three days. Researchers found that one month after the study, the people who used mandalas experienced fewer severe trauma symptoms than those who did not use mandalas (Henderson et al, 2007).

Coloring in mandalas with crayons or colored pencils while spending time in nature is also a relaxing artistic activity and has been shown to reduce chronic pain and stress levels in individuals with chronic widespread musculoskeletal pain (CWP) (Choi et al., 2021).

The International Expressive Arts Therapy Association is a resource for finding local practitioners. https://www.ieata.org/

What are local art resources you would like to share with your clients?

_____

_____

Gratitude Journaling & Cardiovascular Disease

"Calm down or you will end up giving yourself a heart attack" isn't just an old wives' tale. There is a link between stress and cardiovascular disease (CVD). Research suggests that psychological factors, such as chronic stress and depression, are associated with autonomic nervous system (ANS) changes. Moreover, the general consensus is that ANS dysregulation is a predictor of poor CVD outcomes (Redwine et al., 2016).

What can help?

A study on gratitude journaling in clients with asymptomatic Stage B heart failure (HF), found that mindfulness may improve HF morbidity biomarkers, such as inflammation. Thus, mindfulness practices within this important therapeutic window has the potential to slow or stop disease progression, forestalling the development of HF symptoms, and helping maintain quality of life. Researchers also found a relationship between gratitude and inflammatory biomarkers that are linked to adverse cardiac remodeling and progression to HF (Redwine et al., 2016).

What does the practice look like?

The study directed participants that "for the next eight weeks you will be asked to:

- Record 3-5 things for which you are grateful on a daily basis.
- Think back over your day and include anything, however small or great, that was a source of gratitude that day.
- Make the list personal, and try to think of different things each day."

Researchers found that "the average number of journal entries among participants was just over 5 days a week and 89% of participants who started the journaling practice continued to journal for the entire 8 week period." This may be because, according to the researchers, "gratitude journaling requires little equipment, can be performed safely at home, and can be conducted by adult patients of any age with most comorbidities" (Redwine et al., 2016).

Tips for Keeping a Gratitude Journal

- **Be specific** - focus on the details of why and how the things in your life inspire gratitude.

- **Go in depth** - spend a little time focusing on each item in the day's journal entry.

- **Focus on people as well as things** - remember to also focus on people for whom you are grateful.

- **Keep it simple** - you don't need a fancy journal or a timer to start practicing gratitude journaling.

- **Make it a habit** - Set aside a time and place to write in your journal if it's proving hard to adopt as a habit.

- **Don't make it a source of guilt** - feeling gratitude shouldn't feel forced or make you feel guilty or ashamed. Some of us were embarrassed by loved ones and called 'ungrateful' when we tried to advocate for our needs. Gratitude shouldn't feel manipulative.

What are gratitude journaling tips you would like to share with your clients?

_____

_____

IMPORTANT: Journaling may be challenging if the client is blocking out potentially disturbing or overwhelming thoughts. We can offer our clients information about gratitude journaling, but we should never push them to try it.

Coach—Try It Yourself!

If you do not have a meditation practice, challenge yourself to meditate for about ten minutes each day, for about a week.

What did you notice about this experience?

Now try gratitude journaling for about a week.

What did you notice about this experience?

What are lived experiences you would like to share with your clients?

_____

_____

Access to Nature

I invite you to close your eyes for a moment and remember a day where you spent quality time in nature.

- Were you camping, hiking, taking a walk or sitting on a park bench?
- How does spending time in nature make you feel?

If it makes you feel peaceful, happy, and/or relaxed, you are not alone!

In the article, "The Health Benefits of the Great Outdoors: A Systematic Review and Meta-Analysis of Greenspace Exposure and Health Outcomes," researchers found that exposure to greenspace can provide a wide range of health benefits, and greenspace exposure could reduce salivary cortisol, a physiological marker of stress (Twohig-Bennett & Jones, 2018).

Several hypotheses explain the possible relationship between spending time in nature and improved health.

These hypotheses include:

- "Natural and green areas promote health due to the opportunities for physical activity that they present.
- Exercising in a green environment may be more salutogenic than exercising in an indoor gym environment.

- Greenspaces have been associated with social interaction, which can contribute towards improved well-being.
- Sunlight exposure may counteract seasonal affective disorder (SAD), and may be a good source of vitamin D.
- The "old friends" hypothesis, which proposes that use of greenspace increases exposure to a range of microorganisms, including bacteria, protozoa and helminths, which are abundant in nature and may be important for the development of the immune system and for regulation of inflammatory responses.
- Cooling influence of bodies of greenspace on surface radiating temperature (SRT), which has been documented as beneficial for health.
- The mitigation of greenspace against environmental hazards such as air and noise pollution"

(Twohig-Bennett & Jones, 2018)

One type of nature therapy involves using your senses to "experience" a forest. This is called shinrin-yoku ("forest bathing") in Japanese. People who practice shinrin-yoku spend time sitting, lying down, or walking through the forest. Research on forest bathing suggests that phytoncides (volatile organic compounds with antibacterial properties) released by trees may explain the salutogenic properties of shinrin-yoku (Twohig-Bennett & Jones, 2018).

In the article, "Shinrin-Yoku (Forest Bathing) and Nature Therapy: A State-of-the-Art Review," researchers suggest that people exposed to natural greenspaces may experience a reduction in heart rate and blood pressure, and an increase in relaxation. Researchers also found that videos of a forest and/or the ocean may have the same physiological effects. Thus, people who spend time in nature tend to feel safer, calmer, and better overall (Hansen et al., 2017).

Nature is beneficial for children too. Maya Moody, president-elect of the Missouri chapter of the American Academy of Pediatrics, noticed that there have been spikes in childhood anxiety since the arrival of Covid-19. As a result, Moody became one of about a dozen pediatricians who started offering nature-based prescriptions (Biron, 2021).

In the article, "Medical Empirical Research on Forest Bathing (Shinrin-Yoku): A Systematic Review," Wen et al. state that research on the health effects of forest exposure on the human body is gradually increasing. Currently, there are two main mainstream models – forest bathing and horticultural therapy. The forest bathing model encourages both sub-healthy people and sick people to enter the forest for its healing properties. Researchers define "sub-health" as the median between health and disease. The most common symptoms of "sub-health" are fatigue, poor sleep quality, forgetfulness, physical pain, and sore throat. It also includes an increased risk of infection and reduced immune system function (2019).

Horticultural therapy involves guiding sick people to natural environments. The goal of this nature therapy is to treat diseases primarily caused by mental stress (e.g., excessive tension, panic, insomnia, etc.) through social interactions, making crafts, and gardening (Wen et al., 2019).

According to researchers, forest bathing is a type of preventive medicine that is primarily aimed at sub-healthy people, and is focused on preventing disease. Horticultural therapy belongs to the rehabilitation medicine family, which aims to eliminate and reduce dysfunction in the body, and repair and rebuild the body (Wen et al., 2019).

Wen et al. have concluded that the main goal of forest bathing is to experience physical activity or mindfulness practice in nature, using the forest to promote a person's physical and psychological health. Horticultural therapy is focused on hand-to-brain coordination with an emphasis on contact with natural things that promote satisfaction through work. Combining these two has also garnered very good results (2019).

How can we make it safer and easier for our clients to access nature?

Ashley Matheny has a chronic illness and offered great advice at a recent conference for people with lipedema - "if you look for "accessible fishing" you can find areas that are easy to be near the water and often have a bench."

You can find more information on nature therapy here:

- *Accessible Fishing Piers and Platforms*: https://www.access-board.gov/ada/guides/chapter-10-fishing-piers-and-platforms/#accessible-fishing-piers-and-platforms

- *American Horticultural Therapy Association*: https://www.ahta.org/

- *Local Parks:* https://parkrxamerica.org/

- *Improving Urban Health Through Greenspace:* https://www.usda.gov/media/blog/2017/11/28/improving-urban-health-through-green-space

What are local nature resources you would like to share with your clients?

How can we use our "voices," as health experts, to increase the amount of greenspace in our communities?

_____

_____

Coach—Try It Yourself!

Try taking a mindful walk or meditating outdoors - stay curious with your awareness of sound, sight, smell and more.

What did you notice?

What are lived experiences you would like to share with your clients?

Behavioral and Mental Healthcare

It is important to acknowledge that these simple practices are not going to be enough to reduce stress for some clients. Thus, we should refer these clients to professional mental health providers (e.g., psychologists, social workers, counselors, etc.) when necessary.

You can find the National Alliance on Mental Illness (NAMI) guide at https://www.nami.org/Your-Journey/Individuals-with-Mental-Illness/Finding-a-Mental-Health-Professional

Some clients will be optimistic about the initial success they experienced after implementing new habits and behaviors. However, when life gets in the way and stressful situations arise, this progress may derail. Thus, understanding the concept of a window of tolerance could be extremely helpful for our clients.

Concept: "Window of Tolerance" and "Grounding Practices"

"Just Calm Down!"

"Just Get Motivated!"

Have you ever heard two more annoying phrases? Luckily, we have useful tools to teach our clients more than how to "just relax" or "get it done." The first step is accepting that our behavior can change when we experience high arousal levels (frazzled, overstimulated, etc.), moderate levels (focused, balanced, etc.), or low levels of arousal (unmotivated, dissociated, etc.).

Windows of Tolerance and Keeping Your Cool vs. Flying Off the Handle

We are more likely to make good decisions when we are experiencing a moderate level of arousal and are inside our window of tolerance. We are also more likely to feel safe.

Sometimes I can remain calm in a stressful situation and other times I find myself flying off the handle at any little thing. This is because not everyone has the same size 'window' and our 'window size' can change throughout our lives. Having a wider window of tolerance means we can remain at a moderate level of arousal, while experiencing a variety of stressful situations. People with narrow windows of tolerance are typically unable to perform well under pressure, and tend to find it more difficult to stay at a moderate level of arousal during stressful situations.

What is a window of tolerance?

OK, we've described the effects of a window of tolerance, but what is it? In the article, *"War Duration and The Micro-Dynamics of Decision Making Under Stress,"* Stanley describes a window of tolerance as a neurobiological response to stress arousal. This "window" our capability of regulating stress over time to support and elicit optimal performance in the zone of moderate arousal.

What are the benefits of moderate arousal?

Stanley implies that our clients are more likely to do the following inside of their "windows of tolerance:"

- "Engage in an accurate neuroception of opportunity vs. threats
- Synthesize and integrate thinking brain and survival brain processes
- Facilitate concentration and focus
- Facilitate explicit memory formation, consolidation, and retrieval
- Perceive relevant internal and external cues

- Obtain and absorb adequate and appropriate information
- Objectively assess and integrate that information
- Search for all possible options
- Evaluate each option in terms of costs and benefits, by planning and considering the possible future effects
- Choose options that are best aligned with their values and goals"

(Stanley, 2018)

Neff & Germer write about a similar concept in *"The Mindful Self-Compassion Workbook."* The authors state that it is important to allow yourself to go through the process of "opening" and "closing." It is important to be self-compassionate enough to allow yourself to "close" when needed and "open" again when necessary. Signs of "opening" may include laughter, tears, or more vivid thoughts and sensations. Signs of "closing" may include distraction, sleepiness, annoyance, numbness, or self-criticism (2018).

The good news is our current windows of tolerance can *change.* Individual differences in the windows of tolerance are initially wired through the interaction between genetic traits and an early caregiving environment. Childhood stress can result in early-life developmental alterations in one's neurobiological system, leading to a narrow window of tolerance (Stanley, 2018).

Adult experiences can also change windows of tolerance. In other words, adults with normally wide windows of tolerance may find that over time these windows narrow due to chronic stress or trauma (without recovery), or operating a system that is always turned on (never turning it off), such as during stressful decision-making times before and/or during a war (Stanley, 2018). Recovering from stress is an important part of maintaining resilience in the face of repeated stressful situations.

People who work all day at a desk in an office are not shielded from the effects of stress. More specifically, executive functioning may be reduced after high-intensity engagement (e.g., after "cold" cognitive tasks that require detailed attention or "hot" regulatory tasks of modulating stress arousal and negative emotions). This stress arousal may also occur from symbolic or anticipatory threats, and from the recurrence of past traumatic memories (Stanley, 2018).

Knowing this may be helpful for our clients.

Would our clients benefit from practicing stress-reduction techniques immediately after completing cognitive tasks or high stress meetings at work? What practices are they currently using to 'destress'?

Later in the book, we will delve into how to relax after work.

Now, let's look at some practices we can use when we feel hyperaroused or hypoaroused that may bring us back inside our window of tolerance. I call these practices "grounding practices." Before we take a look at them, let's take a moment to recognize times when we feel outside of our window of tolerance.

How can you tell you are outside of your window of tolerance? For me, it's when I notice my inner voice becoming judgemental, fearful, or hypervigilant. I don't have the patience to listen to others and my creativity is stifled.

How do you recognize when you're out of your window of tolerance?

_____

_____

Grounding Practices

The University of Rochester Medical Center's Behavioral Health Partners blog offers a path to reducing anxious thoughts. Researchers suggest that slow, deep, long breaths can help you maintain a sense of calm or help you return to a calmer state.

Once you find your breath, go through the following steps to "ground" yourself:

- Acknowledge **FIVE** things you see around you. It could be a pen, a spot on the ceiling, or anything in your environment.

- Acknowledge **FOUR** things you can touch. It could be your hair, a pillow, or the ground underneath your feet.
- Acknowledge **THREE** things you can hear. It could even be your belly rumbling! You could also focus on things you can hear outside of your body, such a honking horn, barking dog, etc.
- Acknowledge **TWO** things you can smell. It could be the smell of the paper, the ink in your pen, fragrant room spray, flowers, or bathroom soap.
- Acknowledge **ONE** thing you can taste. It could be gum, coffee, or a sandwich. (Smith, 2018).

Here are some more examples of grounding practices that use our senses to allow us to reconnect with our bodies, and provide us a sense of safety and connection:

Sight

- Keep your eyes open during mindfulness
- Search for the colors of the rainbow in your environment
- Look into your pet's or loved one's eyes
- Look at nature scene images (Beukeboom et al., 2012)
- Read poetry (Delamerced et al., 2021) or sacred texts

- Look at icons or photos of saints, or other meaningful art

Sound

- Listen to sounds in your environment
- Listen to soothing music, like the song "Weightless" by Marconi Union (Graff et al., 2019)
- Ask a "safe" person to record a reassuring video or voicemail, and then listen to it
- Listen to binaural beats or 432 Hz music for ten minutes (Menziletoglu et al., 2021; Chaieb et al., 2015; Padmanabhan et al., 2005; Zampi, 2016)
- Listen to birdsong (Zhao et al., 2020)
- Listen to ASMR videos (Eid et al., 2022)

Smell

- Smell essential oils to calm or invigorate you (Farrar & Farrar, 2020)
- Light a scented candle and take in the aroma

Touch

- Feel the sensation of your body against the furniture
- Place one hand over your heart and the other hand on your stomach. Switch hands to see which position is more comfortable

- Try a self-massage. For instance, rub your hands against each other to warm them up, then slide your hands down, starting from your scalp to your face and neck. Next, cross your hands and slide your palms down the opposite shoulder, arm, forearm, and hand
- Self manual lymphatic drainage massage
- Lie under a weighted blanket (Vinson et al. 2020)
- Feel the sensations in your feet
- Stroke a pet or horse (Ein et al., 2018)
- Hold a crystal, amulet, saint card, or something with deep meaning

Thoughts

- Who makes you feel supported – the person who makes you smile when you think of them?
- Think of a "happy place" and focus on the feelings generated in your body

Movement

- Count backwards from twenty as you walk around the room. Pay attention to how your feet feel while walking
- Push against a wall or do wall squats (Morin, n.d.)
- Massage your forearms
- Walk the labyrinth (Davis, 2021; Behman et al., 2018)

- Dance around the room, or "shake it out"
- Doodle on a piece of paper or draw with your hands in the air
- Draw or color mandalas (Henderson et al, 2007; Khodabakhshi-Koolaee, & Darestani-Farahani, 2020) or Zentangle (Hsu et al., 2021)

Breath

- Blow bubbles
- Hum
- Sing
- Breathe in (inhale) and exhale with an audible sigh

Multisensory

- Play computer online/digital games (Collins et al., 2019)
- Embrace indigenous traditions given by elders (Marsh et al., 2015)
- Take a walk outside in nature, especially in a garden with beautiful flowers or herbs
- Wear or hold a loved one's clothing

What are grounding resources you would like to share with your clients?

_____

_____

Coach—Try It Yourself!

Which grounding techniques make sense to you?

Challenge yourself to try them the next time you feel outside your window of tolerance.

What are lived experiences you would like to share with your clients?

_____

_____

PARADIGM SHIFT

Mindfulness may be relaxing for skilled practitioners, but it is not a quick fix that can create instant relaxation after stressful events.

Which activity is best for recovering from a hard day at work?

Some of our clients already have routines that work for them. These individuals' hobbies may include cooking or walking to relax. Other people may turn to wine, cigarettes, and watching television to help them relax.

What can we do if a client has not found a healthy way to recover from a stressful day?

Collins et al. state that four elements must be satisfied to successfully recover from stress:

1. Psychological Detachment (e.g., spending less time thinking about work)
2. Relaxation
3. Mastery (e.g., gaining skills in something other than work)
4. Control (e.g., having control within or over activities)

Researchers have found that online/digital games are more effective at helping people recover from work stress than spending ten minutes learning and practicing mindfulness skills when the mediator is inexperienced (Collins et. al, 2019). Learning mindfulness is hard, and we cannot expect novice meditators to experience mastery or control while they are still learning how to meditate.

Interestingly, researchers also found that mindfulness apps do work well for people coping with hyperarousal. Why? Because "participants appreciated the tiredness that the mindfulness app encouraged as it helped with sleeping or bringing down energy levels when they were unwelcomingly high" (Collins et. al, 2019).

Try the game used in the research study (Block! Hexa Puzzle) here: https://keygames.com/block-hexa-puzzle-game/

The mindfulness intervention studied was the free 5-day beginners' program provided by Headspace.

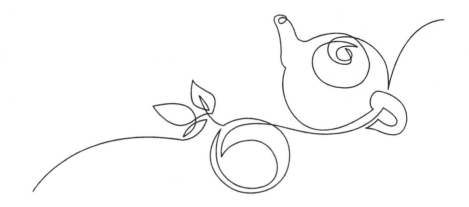

CHAPTER 8

A SELF-CARE TOOLBOX FOR STRESSFUL SITUATIONS

"No plan survives contact with the enemy."
~Famous Military Quote

How many times have we had a big dream that required careful SMART goals, prepped meals, and/or new workout clothes in preparation for a new attitude towards our health – only to have a loved one fall sick, car break down, or the boss hand us a huge new project at work?

We can give ourselves peace of mind simply by having a Plan B and a toolbox for helping us survive stressful situations. Our plans should be flexible enough to withstand and adapt to what life throws at us. If there is one thing life has taught us during the pandemic, it is the importance of self-care during traumatic times.

What are essential tools that your client may need to maintain their health and well-being?

- Access to quality nutrition
- Access to restful sleep
- Access to safe housing
- Access to reliable transportation
- Access to affordable healthcare
- Access to greenspaces
- Opportunities for movement and physical activity
- A consistent schedule
- A sense of community and connection
- Opportunities for self-expression
- Fulfillment of one's life purpose

Many households have emergency kits for natural disasters. These kits may contain canned food, batteries, flashlight, radio, and/or other resources. Invite clients to make an emergency kit or write down a list of tools to use during an emotionally hard time.

This list may contain smartphone relaxation apps with their favorite ones bookmarked, the phone number of a supportive friend or loved one, a book of poems, a journal, a map of local nature trails, calming music, treasured photos, and more.

What are self-care resources you would like to share with your clients?

_____

_____

What experiences drew you to become a mind/ body professional? What are self-care lived experiences you would like to share with your clients?

_____

_____

Helping Clients Reduce Stress Before Surgery

Can we help our clients reduce their stress level before surgery?

Yes! In fact, guided imagery may help. In the article, "Guided Imagery Relaxation Therapy on Preoperative Anxiety: A Randomized Clinical Trial," Felix et al. state that adequately managing preoperative anxiety may improve surgery outcomes, elicit greater patient satisfaction, and decrease hospital costs.

Several mind-body approaches can help alleviate anxiety in people before or during stressful situations, such as with elective surgical procedures. Promising approaches include meditative practices and relaxation techniques that contain guided imagery (Felix et al., 2018).

Preoperative anxiety is associated with problems like difficult venous access, the need for higher doses of anesthetic agents and analgesics, and/or postoperative surgery complications. High levels of anxiety can negatively influence physiological function, and interfere with postoperative recovery, possibly leading to increased hospitalization time (Felix et al., 2018).

Felix et al. also found that guided imagery can effectively reduce anxiety and blood cortisol levels during the preoperative surgery period in patients who were preparing for video laparoscopic bariatric surgeries (2018).

Can an intervention still be effective even if it is not given until after surgery?

My Surgical Success is an online/digital perioperative behavioral pain medicine intervention that is linked to significant acceleration of opioid cessation following surgery (a five-day difference) with no difference in pain levels.

Thus, researchers have concluded that online/digital perioperative behavioral pain medicine may be a low-cost, accessible treatment that supports opioid cessation following breast cancer surgery (Darnall, et al., 2019).

You can find out more about online/digital behavioral pain medicine here: https://bethdarnall.com/blog/2019/05/14/ digital-health-intervention-associated-with-less-need-for-opioids-after-surgery/

Mindful Moment: Shoulder and Neck Rolls

Let's stretch our neck and shoulders for a minute.

Roll your head clockwise three times and counterclockwise three times. Then, roll your shoulders back three times, and forward three times.

How did you feel after taking a short movement break?

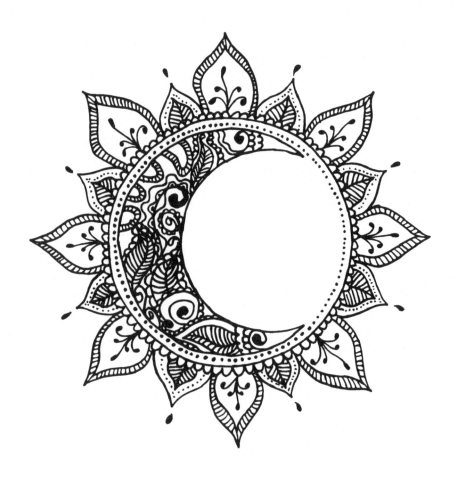

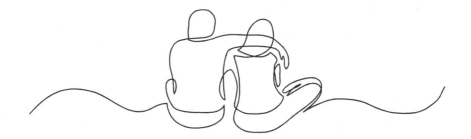

CHAPTER 9
COMMUNITY RESOURCES

What can we do as a community to prevent and reduce the effects of ACEs?

According to the CDC, community risk factors may include communities where neighbors do not know or look out for each other, communities where there is low community involvement among residents, and communities where families frequently experience food insecurity (Risk and Protective Factors, n.d.).

What types of communities are effective at reducing ACEs?

Community protective factors include:

- "Communities with access to safe, stable housing
- Communities where families have access to high-quality preschool
- Communities where families have access to nurturing and safe childcare
- Communities where families have access to safe, engaging after school programs and activities
- Communities where families have access to medical care and mental health services
- Communities where families have access to economic and financial help"

(Risk and Protective Factors, n.d.)

We hold powerful roles as health and wellness experts in the community, and our job is to stand up and speak out for safer communities. I encourage you to volunteer at your local grassroots organizations that seek change in these areas.

Here are some online resources that can help you learn how to successfully prevent and reduce the effects of ACEs in your community:

According to the "ACEs Aware" website, one way to help is by developing cross-sector networks of care within communities and with healthcare teams that are committed to addressing ACEs and toxic stress (For

Communities, n.d.) Find out more here: *Trauma-Informed Network of Care Roadmap:* https://www.acesaware.org/provide-treatment-healing/for-communities/

Paces Connection is a social network that connects people who want to prevent and reduce the impact of ACES in their communities: h t t p s : / / w w w . pacesconnection.com/pages/geographic-communities

How Communities can Foster Resilience (Podcast): https://podcasts.apple.com/us/podcast/roadmap-to-resilience/id1593224431?i=1000542209233

Veterans' Resource

Mindfulness Coach (VA's National Center for PTSD): https://www.ptsd.va.gov/appvid/mobile/mindfulcoach_app.asp

Farm Stress Resource

"12 Tools for Your Wellness Toolbox in Times of Farm Stress" from North Dakota State University: https://www.ag.ndsu.edu/publications/kids-family/12-tools-for-your-wellness-toolbox-in-times-of-farm-stress

Informational Handouts

Informational handouts on reducing toxic stress:

https://www.acesaware.org/wp-content/
uploads/2020/01/Lower-Toxic-Stress-Handout-Adult-
English.pdf

https://www.pacesconnection.com/ws/StressBusters_
General_English.pdf

https://www.pacesconnection.com/ws/StressBusters_
General_Spanish.pdf

What are resources you would like to share with your clients?

_____

_____

Mindful Moment

Place your hand over your heart and feel your heartbeat for 6 breaths.

How did you feel after completing this short exercise? Was it easier to feel your heartbeat toward the end of this exercise?

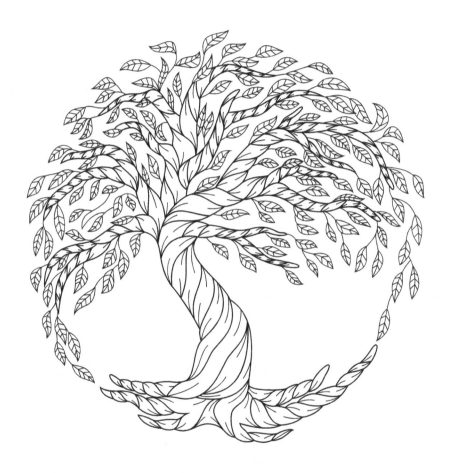

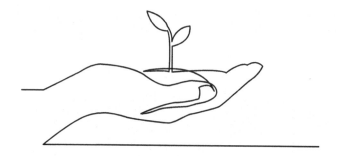

CHAPTER 10
CONCLUSION

Wow! I have shared A LOT of information!

Let's begin this chapter with a mindful moment.

Let's get into a comfortable position, so we can become more aware of our bodies.

I invite you to ask yourself the following questions:

- What prompted me to read this book? What were my goals?
- What out of this book inspired me to learn more?
- What did I learn that will help me better understand my clients?

- Which self-care practices really resonated with me?
- How will I use what I have learned from reading this book in my practice and relationships?

If you like journaling, I invite you to use the questions above as prompts.

_____

_____

_____

My goal is to share the importance of:

- Understanding the impact of ACEs on the mind and body
- Understanding a client's need for safety and how a lack of safety can derail our best efforts at motivational interviewing and providing interventions
- Understanding the **WHY** behind the self-care practices we recommend for our clients
- Encouraging everyone to become the "voice of lived experience" and to try mindful interventions that have been shown to improve resilience
- Encouraging everyone to share these self-care practices with clients, family, and friends

- Encouraging everyone to get involved in their communities to provide equity for all when it comes to access to self-care and thriving communities

Our communities need:

- More public conversations about the negative effects of toxic stress
- More public conversations about self-care
- More access to physical and mental health resources
- More access to safe housing
- More access to nutritious foods
- More access to greenspaces
- More opportunities for community engagement
- More health experts who can effectively spread awareness and reduce the stigma of ACEs

Understand that this mission can only be accomplished through connecting with others and working together as a community, where all voices are heard and honored. Changing or limiting ourselves to fit in is the opposite of truly *belonging*.

Our careers consist of working one-to-one or in small groups with clients who *want* to make a positive change in their health and wellbeing. Our clients will not benefit from a cookie-cutter approach or quick fix that dismisses their lived experiences and their needs for safety and trust.

I hope this book has increased your knowledge and awareness of the effects of ACEs on the mind and body, and raised your confidence in understanding and sharing mindful interventions that can reduce the negative effects of ACEs on our clients' health and wellbeing.

Thank you for all the work you do!

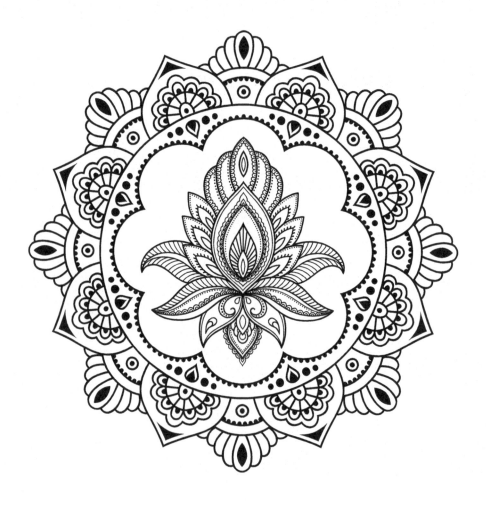

REFERENCES

1. Acabchuk, R. L., Kamath, J., Salamone, J. D., & Johnson, B. T. (2017). Stress and chronic illness: The inflammatory pathway. *Social Science & Medicine, 185*, 166–170. Retrieved from: https://pubmed.ncbi.nlm.nih.gov/28552293/

2. ACEs Aware (2021*). Trauma-informed network of care roadmap.* Retrieved from https://www.acesaware.org/wp-content/uploads/2021/06/Aces-Aware-Network-of-Care-Roadmap.pdf

3. Allen, S. (2018). *The Science of gratitude.* Retrieved from: https://ggsc.berkeley.edu/images/uploads/GGSC-JTF_White_Paper-Gratitude-FINAL.pdf

4. Azam, M. A., Katz, J., Fashler, S. R., Changoor, T., Azargive, S., & Ritvo, P. (2015). Heartrate variability is enhanced in controls but not maladaptive perfectionists during brief mindfulness meditation following stress-induction: A stratified-randomized trial. *Int J Psychophysiology, 98*(1), 27-34. Retrieved from: https://core.ac.uk/download/pdf/77105399.pdf

5. Babatunde, A., Martin, G. C., & Beeson, E. T. (2020). A practitioner's guide to breath work in clinical mental health counseling. *Journal of Mental Health Counseling, 42*(1), 78–94. doi: Retrieved from:https://www.researchgate.net/profile/Babatunde-Aideyan/publication/338569215_A_Practitioner's_Guide_to_Breathwork_in_Clinical_Mental_Health_Counseling/links/5eecf9ab299bf1faac643722/A-Practitioners-Guide-to-Breathwork-in-Clinical-Mental-Health-Counseling.pdf

6. Baker, E., Stover, E., Haar, R., Lampros, A., & Koenig, A. (2020). Safer viewing: A study of secondary trauma mitigation techniques in open source investigations. *Health and Human Rights, 22*(1), 293–304.Retrieved from: https://www.ncbi.nlm.nih.gov/pmc/articles/PMC7348432/

7. Beerse, M. E., Van Lith, T., Pickett, S. M., & Stanwood, G. D. (2020). Biobehavioral utility of mindfulness-based art therapy: Neurobiological underpinnings and mental health impacts. *Exp Biol Med, 245*(2), 122-130. Retrieved from: https://www.ncbi.nlm.nih.gov/pmc/articles/PMC7016419/

8. Behman, P. J., Rash, J. A., Bagshawe, M., & Giesbrecht, J. (2018). Short-term autonomic nervous system and experiential responses during a labyrinth walk. *Cogent Psychology, 5*(1). Retrieved from: https://www.tandfonline.com/doi/full/10.1080/23311908.2018.1495036?src=recsys

9. Beukeboom, C. J., Langeveld, D., & Tanja-Dijkstra, K. (2012). Stress-reducing effects of real and artificial nature in a hospital waiting room. *Journal of Alternative Complementary Medicine, 18*(4):329-33. Retrieved from: https://core.ac.uk/reader/15476039?utm_source=linkout

10. Beutel, M. E., Tibubos, A. N., Klein, E. M., Schmutzer, G., Reiner, I., Kocalevent, R. D., & Brähler, E. (2017). Childhood adversities and distress - The role of resilience in a representative sample. *PloS one, 12*(3). Retrieved from: https://www.ncbi.nlm.nih.gov/pmc/articles/PMC5351992/

11. Biron, C. (2021) *Doctor's orders: 'Nature prescriptions' see rise amid pandemic.* Retrieved from: https://news.trust.org/item/20210831100001-qppwk/

12. Bhushan, D., Kotz, K., McCal,l J., Wirtz, S., Gilgoff, R., Dube, S. R., Powers, C., Olson-Morgan, J., Galeste, M., Patterson, K., Harris, L., Mills, A., Bethell, C., Burke Harris, N. (2020). Roadmap for resilience: The California Surgeon General's report on adverse childhood experiences, toxic stress, and health. *Office of the California Surgeon General.* Retrieved from: https://osg.ca.gov/wp-content/uploads/sites/266/2020/12/Part-II-3.-Tertiary-Prevention-Strategies-in-Healthcare.pdf

13. Brett, F. I., Espeleta, H. C., Lopez, S. V., Leavens, E. L., & Leffingwell, T. R. (2018). Mindfulness as a mediator of the association between adverse childhood experiences and alcohol use and consequences. *Addictive Behaviors, 84*, 92–98. Retrieved from https://doi.org/10.1016/j. addbeh.2018.04.002.

14. Brickel, R. (2017). *Why I take a mind-body approach to trauma recovery.* Retrieved from: https://brickelandassociates.com/ mind-body-approach-trauma-recovery/

15. Brickel, R. (2018). *9 signs you need better self-care and may be a trauma survivor.* Retrieved from: https://brickelandassociates.com/9-signs-you-need-better-self-care-trauma-survivor/

16. Buck, D. W., & Herbst, K. L. (2016). Lipedema: A relatively common disease with extremely common misconceptions. *Plastic and Reconstructive Surgery: Global Open, 4*(9). Retrieved from: https://www.ncbi.nlm.nih.gov/ pmc/articles/PMC5055019/

17. California Surgeon General. (2020). *Report.* Retrieved from: https://osg.ca.gov/sg-report/

18. Chaieb, L., Wilpert, E. C., Reber, T. P., & Fell, J. (2015). Auditory beat stimulation and its effects on cognition and mood States. *Front Psychiatry, 6*(70). Retrieved from: https://www.ncbi.nlm.nih. gov/pmc/articles/PMC4428073/

19. Chaplin, T. M., Niehaus, C., & Gonçalves, S. F. (2018). Stress reactivity and the developmental psychopathology of adolescent substance use. *Neurobiology of Stress, 9*, 133–139. Retrieved from: https://www.ncbi.nlm.nih.gov/pmc/articles/PMC6236512/

20. Chin, B., Lindsay, E. K., Greco, C. M., Brown, K. W., Smyth, J. M., Wright, A., & Creswell, J. D. (2019). Psychological mechanisms driving stress resilience in mindfulness training: A randomized controlled trial. *Health Psychology: Official Journal of the Division of Health Psychology: American Psychological Association, 38*(8), 759–768. Retrieved from: https://www.ncbi.nlm.nih.gov/pmc/articles/PMC6681655/

21. Choi, N., DiNitto, D., Marti, C., & Choi, B. (2017). Association of adverse childhood experiences with lifetime mental and substance use disorders among men and women aged 50 years. *International Psychogeriatrics, 29*(3), 359-372. Retrieved from: https://www.cambridge.org/core/journals/international-psychogeriatrics/article/association-of-adverse-childhood-experiences-with-lifetime-mental-and-substance-use-disorders-among-men-and-women-aged-50-years/0579498316F070E4945E5EA9F1407BE5#

22. Choi H, Hahm SC, Jeon YH, Han JW, Kim SY, Woo JM. The Effects of Mindfulness-Based Mandala Coloring, Made in Nature, on Chronic Widespread Musculoskeletal Pain: Randomized Trial. Healthcare (Basel). 2021 May 28;9(6):642. doi: 10.3390/healthcare9060642. PMID: 34071674; PMCID: PMC8226655. Retrieved from: https://www.ncbi.nlm.nih.gov/pmc/articles/PMC8226655/

23. Cohen, G. L., & Sherman, D. K. (2014). The psychology of change: Self-affirmation and social psychological intervention. *Annual Rev Psychology, 65*, 333-71. Retrieved from: https://pubmed.ncbi.nlm.nih.gov/24405362/

24. Collins, E., Cox, A., Wilcock, C., & Sethu-Jones, G. (2019). Digital games and mindfulness apps: Comparison of effects on post work recovery. *JMIR Ment Health, 6*(7):e12853. Retrieved from: https://www.ncbi.nlm.nih.gov/pmc/articles/PMC6670275/

25. Colloca, L., & Benedetti, F. (2007). Nocebo hyperalgesia: How anxiety is turned into pain. *Current Opinions in Anesthesiology, 20*(5), 435-439. Retrieved from: https://journals.lww.com/co-anesthesiology/Abstract/2007/10000/Nocebo_hyperalgesia__how_anxiety_is_turned_into.7.aspx

26. Cotman, C. W., Berchtold, N. C., & Christie, L. A. (2007). Exercise builds brain health: Key roles of growth factor cascades and inflammation. *Trends in Neuroscience*, *30*(9), 464-72. Retrieved from: https://www.researchgate. net/publication/6075740_Exercise_Builds_ Brain_Health_Key_Roles_of_Growth_Factor_ Cascades_and_Inflammation#fullTextFileContent

27. Darnall, B. D., Sturgeon, J. A., Cook, K. F., Taub, C. J., Roy, A., Burns, J. W., Sullivan, M., & Mackey, S. C. (2017). Development and validation of a daily pain catastrophizing scale. *J Pain*, 18(9), 1139-1149. Retrieved from: https://www.ncbi.nlm. nih.gov/pmc/articles/PMC5581222/

28. Darnall, B. D., & Colloca, L. (2018). Optimizing placebo and minimizing nocebo to reduce pain, catastrophizing, and opioid use: A Review of the science and an evidence-informed clinical toolkit. Int Rev Neurobiology, 139, 129-157. Retrieved from: https://www.ncbi.nlm.nih.gov/pmc/articles/ PMC6175287/

29. Darnall, B. D., Ziadni, M. S., Krishnamurthy, P., Flood, P., Heathcote, L. C., Mackey, I. G., Taub, C. J., & Wheeler, A. (2019). My surgical success: Effect of a digital behavioral pain medicine intervention on time to opioid cessation after breast cancer surgery - A pilot randomized controlled clinical trial. *Pain Medicine, 20*(11), 2228-2237. Retrieved from: https://www.ncbi.nlm.nih.gov/pmc/articles/PMC6830264/

30. Darnall, B. D., Roy, A., Chen, A. L., Ziadni, M. S., Keane, R. T., You, D. S., Slater, K., Poupore-King, H., Mackey, I., Kao, M. C., Cook, K. F., Lorig, K., Zhang, D., Hong, J., Tian, L., & Mackey, S. C. (2021). Comparison of a single-session pain management skills intervention with a single-session health education intervention and 8 sessions of cognitive behavioral therapy in adults with chronic low back pain: A randomized clinical trial. *JAMA network open, 4*(8), e2113401. Retrieved from: https://www.ncbi.nlm.nih.gov/pmc/articles/PMC8369357/

31. Davis, D. W. (2021). A literature review on the physiological and psychological effects of labyrinth walking. *Int J Yogic Hum Mov Sports Sci, 6*(1), 167-175. Retrieved from: https://www.theyogicjournal.com/pdf/2021/vol6issue1/PartC/6-1-61-305.pdf

32. Delamerced, A., Panicker, C., Monteiro, K., & Chung, E. Y. (2021). Effects of a poetry intervention on emotional wellbeing in hospitalized pediatric patients. *Hospital Pediatrics, 11*(3), 263-269. Retrieved from: https://pubmed.ncbi.nlm.nih.gov/33622762/

33. Delude, C. (2015). *Scars that don't fade.* Retrieved from: http://protomag.com/articles/scars-that-dont-fade

34. Dreisoerner, A., Junker, N. M., Schlotz, W., Heimrich, J., Bloemeke, S., Ditzen, B., & van Dick, R. (2021). Self-soothing touch and being hugged reduce cortisol responses to stress: A randomized controlled trial on stress, physical touch, and social identity. *Comprehensive Psychoneuroendocrinology.* Retrieved from: https://www.sciencedirect.com/science/article/pii/S2666497621000655?via%3Dihub&ck_subscriber_id=157723643

35. Eid, C. M., Hamilton, C., Greer, J. M. H. (2022). Untangling the tingle: Investigating the association between the autonomous sensory meridian response (ASMR), neuroticism, and trait & state anxiety. *PLoS One,17*(2), e0262668. Retrieved from: https://www.ncbi.nlm.nih.gov/pmc/articles/PMC8809551/

36. Ein, N, Li, L., & Vickers, K. The effect of pet therapy on the physiological and subjective stress response: A meta-analysis. *Stress Health, 34*(4), 477-489. Retrieved from: https://pubmed. ncbi.nlm.nih.gov/29882342/

37. Farrar, A. J., & Farrar, F. C. (2020). Clinical aromatherapy. *Nurse Clin North Am, 55*(4), 489-504. Retrieved from: https://www.ncbi.nlm.nih. gov/pmc/articles/PMC7520654/

38. Felix, M., Ferreira, M., Oliveira, L. F., Barichello, E., Pires, P., & Barbosa, M. H. (2018). Guided imagery relaxation therapy on preoperative anxiety: A randomized clinical trial. *Revista Latino-Americana de Enfermagem, 26*, e3101. Retrieved from: https://www.ncbi.nlm.nih.gov/ pmc/articles/PMC6280172/

39. For Communities. (n.d.). *Information.* Retrieved from: https://www.acesaware.org/ provide-treatment-healing/for-communities/

40. Franke, H. A. (2014). Toxic stress: Effects, prevention, and treatment. *Children, 1*(3), 390–402. Retrieved from: https://www.ncbi.nlm.nih. gov/pmc/articles/PMC4928741/

41. Frostadottir, A. D., & Dorjee, D. (2019). Effects of mindfulness-based cognitive therapy (MBCT) and compassion-focused therapy (CFT) on symptom change, mindfulness, self-compassion, and rumination in clients with depression, anxiety, and stress. *Frontiers in*

42. *Psychology, 10,* 1099. Retrieved from: https://www.ncbi.nlm.nih.gov/pmc/articles/PMC6534108/

43. Germer, C. K., & Neff, K. (2019). *Teaching the mindful self-compassion program: A guide for professionals.* The Guilford Press.

44. Graff, V., Cai, L., Badiola, I., & Elkassabany, N. M. (2018). Music versus midazolam during preoperative nerve block placements: A prospective randomized controlled study. *Reg Anesth Pain Med*icine. Retrieved from: https://sbgg.org.br/wp-content/uploads/2019/07/1563905859_1_Music_versus_midazolam.pdf

45. Greenwood, B. N., Foley, T. E., Day, H. E., Campisi, J., Hammack, S. H., Campeau, S., Maier, S. F., & Fleshner, M. (2003). Freewheel running prevents learned helplessness/behavioral depression: role of dorsal raphe serotonergic neurons. *The Journal of Neuroscience, 23*(7), 2889–2898. Retrieved from: https://www.jneurosci.org/content/23/7/2889

46. Hansen, M. M., Jones, R., & Tocchini, K. (2017). Shinrin-yoku (forest bathing) and nature therapy: A state-of-the-art review. *Int J Environ Res Public Health, 14*(8), 851. Retrieved from: https://www.ncbi.nlm.nih.gov/pmc/articles/PMC5580555/

47. Henderson, P. G., Rosen, D. H., & Mascaro, N. (2007). Empirical study on the healing nature of mandalas. *Psychology of Aesthetics, Creativity, and the Arts, 1*, 148-154. Retrieved from: https://people.tamu.edu/~David-Rosen/documents/Empirical%20Study%20on%20Healing%20Nature%20of%20Mandalas.pdf

48. Hsu MF, Wang C, Tzou SJ, Pan TC, Tang PL. Effects of Zentangle art workplace health promotion activities on rural healthcare workers. Public Health. 2021 Jul;196:217-222. doi: 10.1016/j.puhe.2021.05.033. Epub 2021 Jul 15. PMID: 34274696. Retrieved from: https://pubmed.ncbi.nlm.nih.gov/34274696/

49. Huberman, A. (2021). *Toolkit for sleep*. Retrieved from: https://hubermanlab.com/toolkit-for-sleep/

50. Jefferson, C. D., Drake, C. L., Scofield, H. M., et al. (2005). Sleep hygiene practices in a population-based sample of insomniacs. *Sleep, 28*(5), 611- 615. Retrieved from https://academic.oup.com/sleep/article/28/5/611/2696899

51. Key Statistics & Graphics. (n.d.). *Information.* Retrieved from: https://www.ers.usda. gov/topics/food-nutrition-assistance/ food-security-in-the-u-s/key-statistics-graphics/

52. Khodabakhshi-Koolaee, A., & Darestani-Farahani, F. (2020). Mandala Coloring as Jungian Art to Reduce Bullying and Increase Social Skills. Retrieved from: https://jccnc.iums.ac.ir/article-1-269-fa.pdf

53. Lindberg, E. (2019). *Practicing gratitude can have profound health benefits, USC experts say.* Retrieved from: https://news.usc.edu/163123/ gratitude-health-research-thanksgiving-usc-experts/

54. Lizier, D. S., Silva-Filho, R., Umada, J., Melo, R., & Neves, A. C. (2018). Effects of reflective labyrinth walking assessed using a questionnaire. *Medicines*, 5(4), 111. Retrieved from: https://www. ncbi.nlm.nih.gov/pmc/articles/PMC6313772/

55. Marsh, T. N., Coholic, D., Cote-Meek, S., et al. (2015). Blending aboriginal and western healing methods to treat intergenerational trauma with substance use disorder in aboriginal peoples who live in northeastern Ontario, Canada. *Harm Reduction Journal, 12*, 14. Retrieved from: https:// harmreductionjournal.biomedcentral.com/ articles/10.1186/s12954-015-0046-1

56. Max Planck Institute for Human Cognitive and Brain Sciences. (2021). Meditation training reduces long-term stress, hair analysis shows. *Science Daily*. Retrieved from: www.sciencedaily.com/releases/2021/10/211007122203.htm

57. McEwen, B. S. (2012). Brain on stress: How the social environment gets under the skin. *Proceedings of the National Academy of Sciences of the United States of America, 109,* 17180–17185. Retrieved from: https://www.ncbi.nlm.nih.gov/pmc/articles/PMC3477378/

58. McKeen, H., Hook, M., Podduturi, P. et al. (2021). Mindfulness as a mediator and moderator in the relationship between adverse childhood experiences and depression. *Current Psychology.* Retrieved from: https://link.springer.com/article/10.1007/s12144-021-02003-z

59. Menziletoglu, D., Guler, A. Y., Cayır, T., & Isik, B. K. (2018). Binaural beats or 432 Hz music? Which method is more effective for reducing preoperative dental anxiety? *Med Oral Patol Oral Cir Bucal, 26*(1):e97-e101. Retrieved from: https://www.ncbi.nlm.nih.gov/pmc/articles/PMC7806348/

60. Mind and Body Practices. (2017). *Information.* Retrieved from: https://www.nccih.nih.gov/health/mind-and-body-practices

61. Morin, A. (n.d.). *Heavy work and sensory processing issues: What you need to* know. Retrieved from: https://www.understood.org/en/articles/heavy-work-activities

62. Naviaux, R. (2021). *Persistent CDR creates blocks in healing that are the shared roots of chronic disease.* Retrieved from: http://naviauxlab.ucsd.edu/science-item/healing-and-recovery/

63. Neff, K. (.n.d.). *Why we need to have compassion for our inner critic.* Retrieved from: https://self-compassion.org/why-we-need-to-have-compassion-for-our-inner-critic/

64. Neff, K., & Germer, C. K. (2018). *The mindful self-compassion workbook: A proven way to accept yourself, build inner strength, and thrive.* Guilford Press.

65. Oleś, P. K., Brinthaupt, T. M., Dier, R., & Polak, D. (2020). Types of inner dialogues and functions of self-talk: Comparisons and implications. *Frontiers in psychology, 11*, 227. Retrieved from: https://www.ncbi.nlm.nih.gov/pmc/articles/PMC7067977/

66. Ortiz, R., & Sibinga, E. M. (2017). The role of mindfulness in reducing the adverse effects of childhood stress and trauma. *Children, 4*(3), 16. Retrieved from: https://www.ncbi.nlm.nih.gov/pmc/articles/PMC5368427/

67. Padmanabhan, R., Hildreth, A. J., & Laws, D. (2005). A prospective, randomized, controlled study examining binaural beat audio and pre-operative anxiety in patients undergoing general anesthesia for day case surgery. *Anesthesia, 60*(9), 874-7. Retrieved from: https://associationofanaesthetists-publications.onlinelibrary.wiley.com/doi/10.1111/j.1365-2044.2005.04287.x

68. Perry, B. D., & Winfrey, O. (2021). *What happened to you? Conversations on trauma, resilience, and healing.* Flatiron Books.

69. Philippus, A., Ketchum, J. M., Payne, L., Hawley, L., & Harrison-Felix, C. (2020). Volunteering and its association with participation and life satisfaction following traumatic brain injury. *Brain injury, 34*(1), 52–61. Retrieved from: https://www.ncbi.nlm.nih.gov/pmc/articles/PMC8552988/

70. Poor Sleep Quality Increases Inflammation, Community Study Finds. (2010). *Information.* Retrieved from: http://shared.web.emory.edu/whsc/news/releases/2010/11/poor-sleep-quality-increases-inflammation-study-finds.html

71. Rani, K., Tiwari, S., Singh, U., Singh, I., & Srivastava N. (2012). Yoga nidra as a complementary treatment of anxiety and depressive symptoms in patients with menstrual disorder. *Int J Yoga, 5*(1), 52-6. Retrieved from: https://www.ncbi.nlm.nih.gov/pmc/articles/PMC3276934/

72. Reid, J. (1972). *Alienation*. Retrieved from: https://www.gla.ac.uk/media/Media_167194_smxx.pdf

73. Redwine, L. S., Henry, B. L., Pung, M. A., Wilson, K., Chinh, K., Knight, B., Jain, S., Rutledge, T., Greenberg, B., Maisel, A., & Mills, P. J. (2016). Pilot randomized study of a gratitude journaling intervention on heart rate variability and inflammatory biomarkers in patients with Stage B heart failure. *Psychosomatic Medicine, 78*(6), 667–676. Retrieved from: https://www.ncbi.nlm.nih.gov/pmc/articles/PMC4927423/

74. Resilience Survey. (n.d.). *Information.* Retrieved from: https://originstraining.org/aces/resilience-survey/

75. Risk and Protective Factors. (n.d.). *Information.* Retrieved from: https://www.cdc.gov/violenceprevention/childabuseandneglect/riskprotectivefactors.html

76. Rivera, A. (2021). *Drop the skirt, how my disability became my superpower.* Amy Rivera & Associates.

77. Shalaby, R., & Agyapong, V. (2020). Peer support in mental health: Literature review. *JMIR mental health, 7*(6), e15572. Retrieved from: https://www.ncbi.nlm.nih.gov/pmc/articles/PMC7312261/

78. Sharpe, E., Lacombe, A., Butler, M. P., Hanes, D., & Bradley R. (2021). A closer look at yoga nidra: Sleep lab protocol. *Int J Yoga Therapy, 31*(1), 20. Retrieved from: https://www.ncbi.nlm.nih.gov/pmc/articles/PMC8932407/

79. Schiraldi, G. R. (2021). *The adverse childhood experiences recovery workbook: Heal the hidden wounds from childhood affecting your adult mental and Physical Health*. New Harbinger Publications, Inc.

80. Schiraldi, G. (2021). *Beginning the healing journey: Return to the resilient zone*. Retrieved from: https://www.psychologytoday.com/us/blog/hidden-wounds/202111/beginning-the-healing-journey-return-the-resilient-zone

81. Schiraldi, G. (2021). *Adverse childhood experiences and emotional intelligence*. Retrieved from: https://www.pacesconnection.com/blog/adverse-childhood-experiences-and-emotional-intelligence

82. Schouten, K. A., de Niet GJ, Knipscheer, J. W., Kleber, R. J., & Hutschemaekers, G. J. (2015). The effectiveness of art therapy in the treatment of traumatized adults: A systematic review on art therapy and trauma. *Trauma Violence Abuse, 16*(2), 220-8. Retrieved from: https://psychotraumanet.org/sites/default/files/documents/Schouten-the%20effectiveness%20of%20art%20therapy%20in%20the%20treatment%20of%20traumatized%20adults.pdf

83. Smith, S. (2018). *5-4-3-2-1 coping technique for anxiety.* Retrieved from: https://www.urmc.rochester.edu/behavioral-health-partners/bhp-blog/april-2018/5-4-3-2-1-coping-technique-for-anxiety.aspx

84. Stanley, E. A. (2018). War duration and the micro-dynamics of decision making under stress. *Polity 50*, 178–200. Retrieved from: https://www.researchgate.net/profile/Elizabeth-Stanley-3/publication/323567624_War_Duration_and_the_Micro-Dynamics_of_Decision_Making_under_Stress/links/5bafee7745851574f7f13f10/War-Duration-and-the-Micro-Dynamics-of-Decision-Making-under-Stress.pdf

85. Talk to your patients and clients about healthy eating routines. (n.d.). *Information.* Retrieved from: https://www.dietaryguidelines.gov/sites/default/files/2021-11/DGA_FactSheet_Clinicians_07-09_508c.pdf

86. Tips for Survivors of a Disaster or other Traumatic Event. (n.d.). *Coping with re-traumatization*. Retrieved from: https://store.samhsa.gov/sites/default/files/d7/priv/sma17-5047.pdf

87. Toxic Stress. (n.d.). *Information*. Retrieved from: https://developingchild.harvard.edu/science/key-concepts/toxic-stress/

88. Treleaven, D. A. (2018). *Trauma-sensitive mindfulness: Practices for safe and transformative healing*. W.W Norton & Company.

89. Twohig-Bennett, C., & Jones, A. (2018). The health benefits of the great outdoors: A systematic review and meta-analysis of greenspace exposure and health outcomes. *Environ Res., 166*, 628-637. Retrieved from: https://www.ncbi.nlm.nih.gov/pmc/articles/PMC6562165/

90. University of Waterloo. (2021). Despite understanding the concept of mindfulness, people are applying it incorrectly, research finds. *Science Daily*. Retrieved from www.sciencedaily.com/releases/2021/11/211108081645.htm

91. Upton, K. V. (2018). An investigation into compassion fatigue and self-compassion in acute medical care hospital nurses: a mixed methods study. *J of Compassionate Health Care* 5, 7. Retrieved from: https://jcompassionatehc.biomedcentral.com/articles/10.1186/s40639-018-0050-x

92. Vaishnav, B. S., Vaishnav, S. B., Vaishnav, V. S., & Varma, J. R. (2011). Effect of yoga-nidra on adolescents' well-being: A mixed method study. *Int J Yoga, 11*(3), 245-248. Retrieved from: https://www.ncbi.nlm.nih.gov/pmc/articles/PMC6134739/

93. Van der Kolk, B. (2014). *The body keeps the score: Mind, brain and body in the transformation of trauma.* Penguin Books.

94. Vinson, J., Powers, J., & Mosesso K. Weighted blankets: Anxiety reduction in adult patients receiving chemotherapy. *Clin J Oncology Nursing, 24*(4), 360-368. Retrieved from: https://pubmed.ncbi.nlm.nih.gov/32678376/

95. Ward, F. (2021). *What is trauma-informed yoga? And, could it actually help us process complex emotions such as grief? Here's what you need to know.* Retrieved from: https://www.glamourmagazine.co.uk/article/what-is-trauma-informed-yoga

96. Wen, Y., Yan, Q., Pan, Y. et al. (2019). Medical empirical research on forest bathing (*Shinrin-yoku*): a systematic review. *Environ Health Prev Medicine, 24*, 70. Retrieved from: https://environhealthprevmed.biomedcentral.com/articles/10.1186/s12199-019-0822-8

97. Williamson, E., Gregory, A., Abrahams, H., Aghtaie, N., Walker, S. J., & Hester, M. (2020). Secondary trauma: Emotional safety in sensitive research. *Journal of Academic Ethics*, *18*(1), 55–70. Retrieved from: https://www.ncbi.nlm.nih.gov/pmc/articles/PMC7223430/

98. Winch, G. (2014). *5 ways to improve your emotional health*. Retrieved from: https://www.psychologytoday.com/us/blog/the-squeaky-wheel/201412/5-ways-improve-your-emotional-health

99. Wood, J. V., Perunovic, W. Q., & Lee, J. W. (2009). Positive self-statements: Power for some, peril for others. *Psychology Science*, *20*(7), 860-6. Retrieved from: https://www.uni-muenster.de/imperia/md/content/psyifp/aeechterhoff/wintersemester2011-12/seminarthemenfelderdersozialpsychologie/04_wood_etal_selfstatements_psychscience2009.pdf

100. Yeung, A., Chan, J. S. M., Cheung, J. C., & Zou, L. (2018). Qigong and tai-chi for mood regulation. *Focus*, *16*(1), 40-47. Retrieved from: https://pubmed.ncbi.nlm.nih.gov/31975898/

101. Xiang, Y., Chao, X., & Ye, Y. (2018). Effect of gratitude on benign and malicious envy: The mediating role of social support. *Front Psychiatry,* *7*(9), 139. Retrieved from: https://www.ncbi.nlm. nih.gov/pmc/articles/PMC5949559/

102. Zampi, D. D. (2016). Efficacy of theta binaural beats for the treatment of chronic pain. *Altern Ther Health Medicine, 22*(1), 32-8.

103. Zhao, W., Li, H., Zhu, X., & Ge, T. (2020). Effect of birdsong soundscape on perceived restorativeness in an Urban Park. *Int J Environ Res Public Health, 17*(16), 5659. Retrieved from: https://www.ncbi.nlm.nih.gov/pmc/articles/ PMC7459586/

104. Zoccola, P. M., & Dickerson, S. S. (2012). Assessing the relationship between rumination and cortisol: A review. *Journal of Psychosomatic Research, 73*(1), 1-9. Retrieved from: https:// www.academia.edu/1255807/Assessing_ the_relationship_between_rumination_and_ cortisol_A_review

Made in USA - Kendallville, IN
48690_9781732806672
11.02.2022 1332